Generalized Anxiety Disorder

Generalized Anxiety Disorder

Symptomatology, Pathogenesis and Management

Edited by

David Nutt DM FRCP FRCPsych FMedSci
Professor of Psychopharmacology
Psychopharmacology Unit
School of Medical Sciences
University of Bristol
Bristol
UK

Karl Rickels MD
Stuart & Emily BH Mudd Professor
Chief, Mood & Anxiety Disorders Section
Department of Psychiatry
University of Pennsylvania Medical Center
Philadelphia, PA
USA

Dan J Stein MD PhD
Director, MRC Unit on Anxiety Disorders
Department of Psychiatry
University of Stellenbosch
Cape Town
South Africa

MARTIN DUNITZ

© 2002 Martin Dunitz Ltd, a member of the Taylor & Francis group

First published in the United Kingdom in 2002
by Martin Dunitz Ltd, The Livery House, 7–9 Pratt Street, London NW1 0AE, UK

Tel: +44 (0) 20 7482 2202
Fax: +44 (0) 20 7267 0159
E-mail: info.dunitz@tandf.co.uk
Website: http://www.dunitz.co.uk

Reprinted 2003

A CIP catalogue record for this book is available from the British Library.

ISBN 1 84184 131 5

Distributed in the USA by
Fulfilment Center
Taylor & Francis
7625 Empire Drive
Florence, KY 41042, USA
Toll Free Tel: +1 800 634 7064
Email: cserve@routledge_ny.com

Distributed in Canada by
Taylor & Francis
74 Rolark Drive
Scarborough, Ontario M1R G2, Canada
Toll Free Tel: +1 877 226 2237
Email: tal_fran@istar.ca

Distributed in the rest of the world by
ITPS Limited
Cheriton House
North Way
Andover, Hampshire SP10 5BE, UK
Tel: +44 (0)1264 332424
Email: salesorder.tandf@thomsonpublishingservices.co.uk

Composition by 𝒯 Tek-Art
Printed and bound in Spain by Grafos S.A. Arte Sobre Papel

Contents

Contributors

Jayne E Bailey
Research Associate
Psychopharmacology Unit
University of Bristol
Bristol
UK

Katja Beesdo Dipl.Psych
Institute of Clinical Psychology and Psychotherapy
Technical University of Dresden
Dresden
Germany

Thomas D Borkovec PhD
Distinguished Professor of Psychology and
Director of Clinical Training
Department of Psychology
The Pennsylvania State University
University Park, PA
USA

Gretchen Carlson MD
Senior Resident in Psychiatry
Department of Psychiatry and Behavioural Sciences
University of Washington School of Medicine
Seattle, WA
USA

Martin Franklin PhD
Assistant Professor
Clinical Director, Center for the Treatment and Study of Anxiety
Department of Psychiatry
University of Pennsylvania
Philadelphia, PA
USA

Ronald C Kessler PhD
Professor, Department of Health Care Policy
Harvard Medical School
Boston, MA
USA

Sarosh Khalid-Khan MD
Postdoctoral Fellow in Clinical Psychopharmacology
Mood and Anxiety Disorders Section
Department of Psychiatry
University of Pennsylvania
Philadelphia, PA
USA

Klaus-Peter Lesch MD
Vice Chair and Professor
Department of Psychiatry and Psychotherapy
University of Würzburg
97080 Würzburg
Germany

Hisato Matsunaga MD PhD
Assistant Professor
Department of Neuropsychiatry
Osaka City Medical School
Osaka
Japan

Susan Mineka PhD
Professor of Psychology and Adjunct Professor of Psychiatry and
Behavioural Sciences
Department of Psychology
Northwestern University
Evanston, IL
USA

David Nutt DM FRCP FRCPsych FMmedSci
Professor of Psychopharmacology
Psychopharmacology Unit
School of Medical Sciences
University of Bristol
Bristol
UK

Suzanne L Pineles MS
Department of Psychology
Northwestern University
Evanston, IL
USA

Ashok Raj MD
Professor of Psychiatry
Department of Psychiatry & Behavioural Medicine
University of Florida
Tampa, FL
USA

Karl Rickels MD
Stuart & Emily BH Mudd Professor of Human Behaviour and
Professor of Psychiatry
Chief, Mood & Anxiety Disorders Section
Department of Psychiatry
University of Pennsylvania Medical Center
Philadelphia, PA
USA

Peter P Roy-Byrne MD
Professor and Vice Chair
Department of Psychiatry and Behavioural Sciences
University of Washington School of Medicine and Chief of Psychiatry
Harborview Medical Center
Seattle, WA
USA

Moira A Rynn MD
Assistant Professor of Psychiatry
Medical Director, Mood and Anxiety Disorders Section
Department of Psychiatry
University of Pennsylvania
Philadelphia, PA
USA

David V Sheehan MD MBA
Professor and Director of Research
Department of Psychiatry & Behavioural Medicine
University of South Florida
Tampa, FL
USA

Melinda A Stanley PhD
Professor, Department of Psychiatry and Behavioural Sciences
University of Texas – Houston Health Science Center
Houston, TX
USA

Dan J Stein MD PhD
Director, MRC Unit on Anxiety Disorders
Department of Psychiatry
University of Stellenbosch
Cape Town
South Africa

Hans-Ulrich Wittchen PhD
Professor, Institute of Clinical Psychology and Psychotherapy
Technical University of Dresden and
Max Planck Institute of Psychiatry
Muenchen
Germany

Iftah Yovel MS
Department of Psychology
Northwestern University
Evanston, IL
USA

Preface

Chronic anxiety has long been recognized as an important clinical problem in both specialist settings and in primary care. Nevertheless, the introduction of generalized anxiety disorder into the formal diagnostic nomenclature was marred by its initial conceptualization as a residual diagnostic category. Furthermore, early research on GAD was similarly interpreted as showing that this was not an independent disorder, but rather a residual condition, a prodrome, or a severity marker.

Advances in research on GAD, however, established that this disorder is an important independent condition; one that is prevalent, chronic, and disabling. Thus, for example, GAD is the most common anxiety disorder in primary care, and in an important recent survey it was found to be the most impairing of more than 12 general medical and psychiatric conditions. This volume aims in part to highlight this new understanding of GAD.

We believe that a volume on GAD is particularly timely in view of the broad range of recent progress in understanding the psychobiology and management of this disorder. Such progress has taken place on a broad range of fronts; there has been increased recognition of GAD in different populations (e.g., adolescents and the elderly), in understanding neurobiological and psychological mechanisms underlying GAD, and in the pharmacotherapy and psychotherapy of this disorder.

This volume aims to provide clinicians with an up-to-date review of GAD. Leading authorities from around the world concurred that a review of GAD was timely, and kindly agreed to provide chapters that would synthesize research and be useful in the clinic. The resulting volume comprehensively covers the symptomatology, pathogenesis, and treatment of GAD. We would like to record our thanks for these wonderful contributions, and our gratitude to Ruth Dunitz and her team for making this book happen.

Editors
2002

I   Symptoms

1

Evidence that Generalized Anxiety Disorder is an Independent Disorder

Ronald C Kessler

The notion of persistent pathological anxiety has been a central concept in psychiatry since the founding of the discipline in the nineteenth century. Yet the American Psychiatric Association (APA) did not introduce the diagnosis of generalized anxiety disorder (GAD) into their Diagnostic and Statistical Manual of Mental Disorders (DSM) until the 1980 publication of the third edition.[1] The World Health Organization (WHO) only introduced the diagnosis of GAD into the International Classification of Diseases in the 1990 tenth edition.[2] Before these changes, GAD was conceptualized as one of the two main components of anxiety neurosis, the other component being panic. Recognition that these two syndromes are sufficiently independent to be considered distinct disorders led to the separation of panic and GAD in DSM-III and ICD-10. However, both of these diagnostic systems, but especially DSM-III, conceptualized GAD as a residual diagnosis and considered the clinical significance of GAD as fairly minor.

The DSM-III definition of GAD required uncontrollable and diffuse (i.e., not focused on a single major life problem) anxiety or worry that was excessive or unrealistic in relation to objective life circumstances and that persisted for one month or longer. A number of psychophysiological symptoms were required to occur with the anxiety or worry. Early studies that evaluated DSM-III GAD in clinical samples found that the disorder seldom occurred in the absence of some other comorbid anxiety or mood disorder and that there was an especially strong relationship of GAD with major depression.[3,4] This led some commentators to suggest that GAD might better be conceptualized as a prodrome, residual, or severity marker of depression rather than as an independent disorder.[5,6,7]

As comorbidity between GAD and depression was found to be lower when the duration of GAD increased,[8] the DSM-III-Revised (DSM-III-R) committee changed the one-month minimum duration requirement of GAD to six months.[9] This same duration requirement was used in ICD-10[2] and was retained in DSM-IV.[10] ICD-10 and DSM-IV also changed some of the DSM-III symptom requirements for psychophysiological symptoms associated with persistent and diffuse worry and anxiety in an effort to remove some of the symptoms that are also frequently found among people with depression.

Clinical studies using DSM-III-R criteria found that comorbidity remained quite high even with the six-month duration requirement.[7,11] This led to continued suggestions that GAD is not an independent disorder, but rather a prodrome, residual, or severity marker of depression.[12,13] Despite these suggestions, though, the current view is that GAD is an independent disorder. This view is based on five types of evidence that are reviewed in this chapter: (1) that there is meaningful symptom specificity of GAD in relation to major depression; (2) that GAD is not more highly comorbid than other anxiety and mood disorders in general population samples; (3) that the predictors of GAD are quite different from the predictors of depression; (4) that the course of GAD is more independent of comorbidity than the course of other anxiety or mood disorders; and (5) that the impairments associated with pure GAD are comparable to those associated with other pure anxiety and mood disorders. Each of these five bodies of evidence is reviewed in successive sections of this chapter. The chapter closes with a brief discussion of remaining uncertainties and suggestions for future investigation.

Symptom specificity

An issue of special importance in the evaluation of comorbidity is whether the symptoms of a presumably distinct disorder form separate empirical clusters from symptoms of other disorders in representative clinic and community samples.[14] This is especially important for GAD in that some of the psychophysiological symptoms of the disorder specified in the DSM-III and DSM-III-R definitions overlap with the symptoms of major depression. As noted above, this overlap was reduced in the modification of the diagnostic criteria in DSM-IV. However, some overlap still remains. An important question, then, is whether the high comorbidity of GAD with depression is due to conceptual confounding that might be reduced by further modifications of the diagnostic criteria.

Maier and his colleagues[15] evaluated this issue in the WHO study on psychological problems in primary care by analysing retrospective reports obtained in a survey of patients regarding the frequency of anxiety-mood spectrum symptoms during the 30 days before the interview. Their question was whether the psychophysiological symptoms stipulated for GAD in ICD-10 cluster with the core symptoms of GAD (i.e., persistent worry and anxiety), with the core symptoms of depression (i.e., dysphoria and anhedonia), or with both sets of core symptoms. Their analysis showed clearly that these psychophysiological symptoms cluster strongly only with the core symptoms of GAD.

Brown, Chorpita, and Barlow[16] carried out a more extensive psychometric investigation along the same lines as Maier et al. that tested several models of structural relationships among all the symptoms of GAD and major depression in a mixed treatment sample. They found separate latent factors of positive affectivity, negative affectivity, and autonomic suppression that largely explained the clustering among these symptoms. Patients with GAD were found to have high elevation in the cluster of autonomic suppression, while patients with depression did not, showing that the multivariate symptom profiles characteristic of GAD and major depression can be distinguished despite the overlap of some core symptoms.

Comorbidity

The early evidence of high comorbidity in GAD that was reviewed in the introduction came almost entirely from clinical samples. Studies of GAD comorbidity carried out in community samples suggest that the initial concern about extremely high comorbidity in GAD was misplaced. Wittchen et al.[17] first documented this in an analysis of a large community epidemiological survey, which showed that the proportion of people with DSM-III-R GAD and one or more other comorbid diagnoses is not dramatically higher than the rate of comorbidity among people with other anxiety or mood disorders. Wittchen and his colleagues showed that the discrepancy between this result and earlier clinical findings of much more comorbidity in GAD than in other disorders is due to the fact that comorbidity is a powerful predictor of help-seeking among people with GAD. This suggests that the extremely high comorbidity in GAD is an artifact of treatment sample selection bias rather than an inherent feature of GAD. Kessler et al.[18] subsequently replicated the Wittchen et al. findings in a series of epidemiological surveys carried out in a number of different countries.

Differential predictors of GAD and depression

Another piece of evidence that argues for the independence of GAD, especially from major depression, is that epidemiological surveys show consistently that GAD and major depression have significantly different sociodemographic predictors.[19] For example, socioeconomic status is much more strongly related to major depression than to GAD.

Studies of stressful life events also show that the provoking events that lead to GAD are quite different from those that lead to depression,[20,21] with loss events leading to depression and danger events (i.e., events that create the possibility of future loss) leading to GAD. Analyses of twin data using an additive behavior genetic model also conclude that the environmental determinants of GAD and major depression are distinct.[22]

One seemingly contradictory piece of evidence regarding the different predictors of GAD and depression comes from twin studies, which suggest that the genes for GAD and major depression are the same.[22] This raises the possibility that the two syndromes are different manifestations of the same underlying disorder. However, the model on which this conclusion is based assumes that the joint effects of genes and environment are additive; that is, that the impact of environmental determinants is not influenced by the presence or absence of genes. This is implausible. A more realistic interactive specification, which cannot be identified with conventional twin data, might well show differentiation of genetic effects. Consistent with this possibility, family studies show differential aggregation of mental disorders in the families of patients with GAD and major depression.[23] This observation has been used to argue against the evidence from twin studies to suggest that GAD and major depression are distinct disorders at a genetic level.[24]

Predictive priorities in lifetime comorbid GAD

A more direct way to study predictive differences in GAD compared to other anxiety and mood disorders is to investigate whether one disorder in a particular comorbid pair, when it is temporally primary, is a significant predictor of the subsequent first onset of the other disorder. This was first examined by Kessler[25] in an analysis of data from the U.S. National Comorbidity Survey (NCS). Retrospective age-at-onset reports for each disorder assessed in the NCS were used to estimate a series of bivariate survival models in which prior onset of one disorder was treated as a time-varying covariate of each of the other disorders assessed in the survey. All temporally primary anxiety and mood disorders were found to be statistically significant predictors of the subsequent first onset of other anxiety and mood disorders. GAD did not stand out in any particular way in comparison to the other disorders either in the magnitude of the effects of GAD in predicting later onset of other disorders or in the magnitude of the effects of other temporally primary disorders in predicting first onset of GAD.

This pattern of results was subsequently replicated in a series of epidemiological surveys carried out in a number of different countries.[18] These same cross-national data were also used to investigate whether comorbidity is associated more strongly with the severity or course of GAD than other anxiety or mood disorders.[18] The rationale was that, if GAD is a prodrome, residual, or severity marker of other disorders, the severity and course of GAD would be much more strongly affected by comorbidity than would the severity and course of other anxiety or mood disorders. Although the results showed that comorbidity is generally associated with increased severity and persistence for all anxiety and mood disorders, a very important difference was found for GAD: GAD was the only anxiety or mood disorder in which persistence, as indirectly indicated by recency controlling for age at onset and time since onset, was unrelated to comorbidity.

Yonkers et al.[26] reported the same result in an analysis of the prospective predictors of the clinical course of GAD in the Harvard-Brown Anxiety Research Program (HARP), in which the course of comorbid GAD was found to be unrelated to whether the GAD is primary or secondary.[27] Although some other studies have arrived at different conclusions about the effects of comorbidity on the course of GAD,[28,29,30] the inconsistency of this evidence in conjunction with the clear and consistent evidence that comorbidity is significantly related to the course of other anxiety and mood disorders means that, if anything, GAD behaves more like an independent disorder in this respect than do other anxiety or mood disorders.

The impairments associated with pure and comorbid GAD

As previously noted, Wittchen and his associates found that the false appearance of high comorbidity in GAD in early clinical studies is due to an exceptionally strong help-seeking bias among people with comorbid GAD. People in the general population with GAD had extremely low rates of help-seeking for GAD in the absence of some other comorbid mental disorder. There are at least two plausible interpretations of this finding. One is that pure GAD is not seriously impairing in itself; only when GAD co-occurs with other anxiety or mood disorders does the level of distress in GAD motivate people with the disorder to seek treatment. If this is the case, it could be argued that GAD may be an independent disorder, but it is only clinically significant when it is part of a comorbid cluster in which the comorbid disorders should be the focus of clinical attention. The other plausible interpretation is that people with GAD worry about a great many things, but seldom perceive that their worrying is a problem without the presence of other comorbid disorders more easily recognized as pathological. The distinction between these two possibilities is of considerable importance in evaluating whether GAD should be considered a clinically significant disorder in its own right.

A number of recent studies have compared these two possibilities in primary care samples[31,32,33] and general population samples.[34,35] The results of these studies are reviewed (see Chapter 2) and are consequently not discussed here other than to note that the findings consistently show that pure GAD is equally, if not more, impairing than other pure anxiety and mood disorders. This means that the low rate of treatment for pure GAD is not due to pure GAD being a clinically insignificant disorder. Several other recent studies have presented suggestive evidence that people with pure GAD, despite their impairments, usually fail to seek help because they do not recognize themselves as having an emotional problem.[36]

Overview

The weight of evidence reviewed in this chapter argues strongly that GAD is an independent disorder rather than a prodrome, residual, or severity marker of depression or of some other anxiety or mood disorder. Yet it is also clear that the strong comorbidities found among the anxiety and mood disorders imply that there are either important common causes of these disorders or that some of these disorders cause others. As the available evidence

suggests that GAD is more often than not a primary disorder when it is involved in these comorbidities, it would be useful for future research to evaluate the impact of GAD on the onset and course of other disorders.

With regard to onset, the evidence is clear that temporally primary GAD significantly strongly predicts the subsequent first onset of depression and other secondary disorders. A question can consequently be raised whether early intervention and treatment of primary GAD might be effective in preventing the subsequent first onset of secondary depression. We do not know the answer to this question because, as discussed earlier in the chapter, people with pure GAD seldom seek treatment. However, given the high prevalence, significant impairment, and risk of secondary disorders associated with pure GAD, outreach efforts aimed at encouraging treatment among people with pure GAD are clearly warranted. Effectiveness trials that evaluate whether treatment of pure GAD reduces risk of subsequent secondary disorders would also be of great value.

An issue of considerable importance in designing such interventions is that the current ICD and DSM definitions of GAD are probably too narrow, which means that the number of people eligible for early outreach and treatment of primary GAD is probably a good deal larger than one might expect based on GAD prevalence estimates. As reviewed by Rickels et al (see Chapter 3), there are many people with a GAD-like syndrome who experience clinically significant distress and impairment but never have episodes that last as long as six months. It is unclear whether these people have the same elevated risk of secondary depression as those who meet ICD or DSM criteria of GAD. Naturalistic longitudinal studies that begin with a sample of young people who are followed over many years are needed to investigate this issue and to help target early interventions.

With regard to course, the evidence is clear that GAD is usually more persistent than other comorbid disorders. The hierarchy rules in DSM-IV retain a residual of the biased initial thinking about GAD in the stipulation that a diagnosis of GAD cannot be made if the anxiety occurs exclusively within an episode of major depression. This stipulation is of little practical importance because the number of people with GAD whose anxiety occurs exclusively within episodes of major depression is quite small. However, a sizable number of people have episodes of major depression that occur exclusively within longer episodes of anxiety. Yet DSM-IV has no symmetric hierarchy rule that these episodes of depression do not qualify for a diagnosis of major depression.

This frequent occurrence of depression within longer episodes of GAD, as described in the evidence reviewed in this chapter, is associated with a more persistent course of major depression (although not of GAD). It would be useful for future clinical and epidemiological studies to investigate the implications of this observation. One such implication is that different treatment strategies might prove to be effective in resolving depressive episodes in the presence versus the absence of comorbid GAD. We know that

comorbid GAD is a significant predictor of treatment resistance among patients in treatment for depression.[37] We do not know, though, whether optimal treatment strategies vary depending on whether depression occurs with or without comorbid GAD. Another implication is that maintenance treatment for patients with resolved episodes of depression might be more necessary if their depression occurs in conjunction with GAD. We know that maintenance medication reduces risk of depression relapse.[38] We do not know, though, whether this effect varies depending on whether the patient has a history of GAD or perhaps has unremitted GAD at the time of the remission of the index depressive episode.

Acknowledgements

Preparation of this chapter was supported by U.S. Public Health Service grant U01-MH60220 and by the Global Research on Anxiety and Depression Network (GRAD; www.gradnetwork.com). GRAD is supported by an unrestricted educational grant from Wyeth-Ayerst Pharmaceuticals. The helpful comments of Sergio Aguilar-Gaxiola, Kathleen Merikangas, Bedirhan Ustun, and Hans-Ulrich Wittchen are gratefully acknowledged.

References

1. American Psychiatric Association, *Diagnostic and Statistical Manual of Mental Disorders: DSM-III*, 3rd edn (American Psychiatric Association: Washington, DC, 1980).

2. World Health Organization, *The International Classification of Diseases, 10th revision – Classification of mental and behavioral disorders: Diagnostic criteria for research* (World Health Organization: Geneva, 1990).

3. Breier A, Charney DS, Heninger GR, The diagnostic validity of anxiety disorders and their relationship to depressive illness, *Am J Psychiatry* (1985) 142:787–97.

4. Breslau N, Depressive symptoms, major depression and generalized anxiety: a comparison of self-reports on CES-D and results from diagnostic interviews, *Psychiatry Res* (1985) 15:219–29.

5. Breslau N, Davis GC, Further evidence on the doubtful validity of generalized anxiety disorder, *Psychiatry Res* (1985) 16:177–9.

6. Clayton PJ, Grove WM, Coryell W, Keller MB, Hirschfeld R, Fawcett J, Follow-up and family study of anxious depression, *Am J Psychiatry* (1991) 148:1512–7.

7. Noyes R Jr, Woodman C, Garvey MJ, Cook BL, Suelzer M, Clancy J, Anderson DJ, Generalized anxiety disorder vs. panic disorder. Distinguishing characteristics and patterns of comorbidity, *J Nerv Ment Dis* (1992) 180:369–79.

8. Breslau N, Davis GC, DSM-III generalized anxiety disorder: An empirical investigation of more stringent criteria, *Psychiatry Res* (1985) 15:231–8.

9. American Psychiatric Association, *Diagnostic and Statistical Manual of Mental Disorders: DSM-III-R*, 3rd edn-rev (American Psychiatric Association: Washington, DC, 1987).

10 American Psychiatric Association, *Diagnostic and Statistical Manual of Mental Disorders: DSM-IV*, 4th edn (American Psychiatric Association: Washington, DC, 1994).

11 Roy-Byrne PP, Generalized anxiety and mixed anxiety-depression: Association with disability and health care utilization, *J Clin Psychiatry* (1996) 57:86–91.

12 Brawman-Mintzer O, Lydiard RB, Emmanuel N, Payeur R, Johnson M, Roberts J, Jarrell MP, Ballenger JC, Psychiatric comorbidity in patients with generalized anxiety disorder, *Am J Psychiatry* (1993) 150:1216–8.

13. Gorman JM, Comorbid depression and anxiety spectrum disorders, *Depress Anxiety* (1996) 4:160–8.

14. Robins E, Guze SB, Establishment of diagnostic validity in psychiatric illness: Its application to schizophrenia, *Am J Psychiatry* (1970) 126:983–7.

15. Maier W, Gansicke M, Freyberger HJ, Linz M, Heun R, Lecrubier Y, Generalized anxiety disorder (ICD-10) in primary care from a cross-cultural perspective: A valid diagnostic entity?, *Acta Psychiatr Scand* (2000) 101:29–36.

16. Brown TA, Chorpita BF, Barlow DH, Structural relationships among dimensions of the DSM-IV anxiety and mood disorders and dimensions of negative affect, positive affect, and autonomic arousal, *J Abnorm Psychol* (1998) 107:179–92.

17. Wittchen H-U, Zhao S, Kessler RC, Eaton WW, DSM-III-R generalized anxiety disorder in the National Comorbidity Survey, *Arch Gen Psychiatry* (1994) 51:355–64.

18. Kessler RC, Andrade LH, Bijl RV, Offord DR, Demler OV, Stein DJ, The effects of comorbidity on the onset and persistence of generalized anxiety disorder in the ICPE surveys *Psychol Med* (in press).

19. Skodal AE, Schwartz S, Dohrenwend BP, Levav I, Shrout PE, Minor depression in a cohort of young adults in Israel, *Arch Gen Psychiatry* (1994) 51:542–51.

20. Finlay-Jones R, Brown GW, Types of stressful life event and the onset of anxiety and depressive disorders, *Psychol Med* (1981) 11:803–15.

21. Finlay-Jones R, Anxiety. In: Brown GW, Harris TO, eds, *Life Events and Illness* (Guildford Press: New York, 1989) 95–112.

22. Kendler KS, Neale MC, Kessler RC, Heath AC, Eaves LJ, Major depression and generalized anxiety disorder: Same genes, (partly) different environments?, *Arch Gen Psychiatry* (1992) 49:716–22.

23. Reich J, Distinguished mixed anxiety/depression from anxiety and depressive groups using the family history method, *Compr Psychiatry* (1993) 34:285–90.

24. Reich J, Family psychiatric histories in male patients with generalized anxiety disorder and major depressive disorder, *Ann Clin Psychiatry* (1995) 7:71–8.

25. Kessler RC, The prevalence of psychiatric comorbidity. In Wetzler S, Sanderson WC, eds, *Treatment strategies for patients with psychiatric comorbidity* (John Wiley & Sons: New York, 1997) 23–48.

26. Yonkers KA, Dyck IR, Warshaw M, Keller MB, Factors predicting the clinical course of generalised anxiety disorder, *Br J Psychiatry* (2000) 176:544–9.

27. Rogers MP, Warshaw MG, Goisman RM, Goldenberg I, Rodriguez-Villa F, Mallya G, Freeman SA, Keller MB, Comparing primary and secondary generalized anxiety disorder in a long-term naturalistic study of anxiety disorders, *Depress Anxiety* (1999) 10:1–7.

28. Angst J, Vollrath M, The natural history of anxiety disorder and generalized anxiety disorder, *Acta Psychiatrica* (1991) 141:572–5.

29. Durham RC, Allan T, Hackett CA, On predicting improvement and relapse in generalized anxiety disorder following psychotherapy, *Br J Clin Psychol* (1997) 36:101–19.

30. Mancuso DM, Townsend MH, Mercante DE, Long-term follow-up of generalized anxiety disorder, *Compr Psychiatry* (1993) 34:441–6.

31. Olfson M, Fireman B, Weissman MM, Leon AC, Sheehan DV, Kathol RG, Hoven C, Farber L, Mental disorders and disability among patients in a primary care group practice, *Am J Psychiatry* (1997) 154:1734–40.

32. Ormel J, Von Korff M, Ustun B, Pini S, Korten A, Oldehinkel T, Common mental disorders and disability across cultures: Results from the WHO collaborative study on psychological problems in general health care, *J Am Med Assoc* (1994) 272:1741–8.

33. Schonfeld WH, Verboncoeur CJ, Fifer SK, Lipschutz RC, Lubeck DP, Bueschinf DP, The functioning and well-being of patients with unrecognized anxiety disorders and major depressive disorder, *J Affect Disord* (1997) 43:105–19.

34. Kessler RC, Dupont RL, Berglund P, Wittchen H-U, Impairments of twelve-month independent and comorbid generalized anxiety disorder and major depression in two national surveys, *Am J Psychiatry* (1999) 156:1915–23.

35. Wittchen H-U, Mueller N, Storz S, Psychische Stoerungen: Haufigkeit, psychosoziale Beeintraechtigungen und Zusammenhaenge mit koerperlichen Erkrankungen, *Das Gesundheitswesen* (1998) 60 Sonderheft 2:s95–100.

36. Olfson M, Kessler RC, Berglund PA, Lin E, Psychiatric disorder onset and first treatment contact in the United States and Ontario, *Am J Psychiatry* (1998) 155:1415–22.

37. Petersen T, Gordon JA, Kant A, Fava M, Rosenbaum JF, Nierenberg AA, Treatment resistant depression and Axis I co-morbidity, *Psychol Med* (2001) 31:1223–9.

38. Kupfer DJ, Frank E, Perel JM, Cornes C, Mallinger AG, Thase ME, McEachran AB, Grochocinski VJ, Five-year outcome for maintenance therapies in recurrent depression, *Arch Gen Psychiatry* (1992) 49:769–73.

2

The Impact of Generalized Anxiety Disorder

Hans-Ulrich Wittchen, Katja Beesdo and Ronald C Kessler

Introduction

Over the past decade there has been a growing interest in understanding the nosological status, clinical implications, and public health importance of generalized anxiety disorder (GAD). Much of this interest has been fuelled by the growing recognition that patients with GAD are highly prevalent in primary care, that they cause significant burden to primary care doctors because of their frequent presentation for treatment of vaguely defined physical complaints, and that the underlying anxiety that presumably leads to this high utilization of primary care services is only seldom recognized by the primary care doctors who treat them.[1,2] Increasing availability of new psychological and pharmacological treatments has added to the interest in these observations.[3,4]

Parallel to the growing interest in GAD in primary care, there has also been a growth in broader studies of GAD in the community. These studies have moved from initial investigations of prevalence (e.g., Wittchen et al.[5]) to more recent efforts to examine the total burden associated with GAD (e.g., Kessler, Keller & Wittchen[6]). The most recent studies of this sort have attempted to provide detailed descriptions of GAD-specific impairments and disabilities and the quality of life of people with GAD. In addition, some attempts have been made in these studies to derive crude estimates of the economic burden of GAD.

The development of the above studies lagged behind similar investigations of other mental disorders because of concerns about the independent nosological status of GAD. These concerns are based on the findings of low diagnostic reliability for GAD as defined by DSM-III-R criteria[7,8] and the observation that GAD seems to be usually comorbid with other disorders and rarely presents in clinical settings in its pure form.[5,9,10] Recent progress in the development of reliable diagnostic criteria and instruments has now resolved most of these concerns. Changes in diagnostic criteria in DSM-IV removed the least reliable aspects of the GAD diagnosis, while detailed explorations of comorbidity in the community showed that the proportion of comorbidity among DSM-III-R GAD sufferers does not differ significantly from proportions of comorbidity in most other anxiety and affective disorders (see Chapter 1).[11] Arguments against the validity of GAD have waned as a result.

One important step in establishing the nosological status of GAD is to demonstrate that there are impairments, disabilities and reductions in quality of life that are specifically associated with this disorder rather than with comorbid conditions. An additional step is to demonstrate the importance of GAD within a public health perspective in terms of its prediction of health-care utilization patterns, as well as its economic impact. These types of questions are of relevance to all public health workers. Clinicians need to become aware of the acute and long-term adverse life consequences of unresolved GAD and to adopt appropriate pharmacological and psychosocial interventions in order to compensate for existing disabilities during their treatment strategies.

Impairments and disabilities of GAD

Several research approaches have specifically examined the impairments and disabilities of GAD, including clinical studies, studies in primary care settings, and studies of general population surveys. Despite considerable variability with regard to sampling of cases and patients, diagnostic standards and systems, and types of measures used to quantify impairment and disability, there is good agreement across these studies regarding the frequency and types of impairment and disabilities typically associated with GAD.

Primary care studies

Three primary care studies found that pure GAD, defined as a current episode of GAD in the absence of any of the other mood, anxiety, or substance-use disorders, was associated with meaningful levels of impairment in several life domains. In the largest of these studies, Ormel et al.[12] found that mean numbers of disability days in the past month were much higher among primary care patients with pure GAD (4.4 days) than among patients with none of the psychiatric disorders assessed in their survey (1.7 days). This study included n=272 pure ICD-10 GAD cases and further revealed that non-comorbid GAD had higher occupational role dysfunctions, and higher self-reported physical disability scores. Additionally, in this study, disability outcomes were similar for pure GAD and pure depression.

Schonfeld et al.[13] found that mean age-adjusted and sex-adjusted scores on the 0–100 Short-Form Health Survey (SF-36) scale of social functioning[14] were much lower (with a high score indicating good functioning) among primary care patients with pure GAD (score, 71.0) than among patients with none of the psychiatric disorders assessed in their primary care survey (score, 83.6). They also suggested that DSM-III-R GAD led to lower scores for several areas of functioning, but the negative impact of non-comorbid GAD was not as great as the negative impact of non-comorbid major depression.[13] Differences in the magnitude of impairment associated with pure GAD versus pure depression were much smaller in the study by Ormel et al.,[12] which included many more respondents with pure GAD (n=272) and pure depression (n=438). Aggregate impairments of GAD and major depression were also found to be similar to each other in a large primary care study conducted by Spitzer et al.[15] that did not, however, distinguish between pure and comorbid cases.

An exception to the general pattern of finding significant impairments in pure GAD is a small study by Olfson et al.,[16] which found that DSM-IV GAD was only associated with significant disability if it was comorbid. However, the reliability of this finding can be called into question based on the fact that there were only 14 patients with pure GAD in this sample.

These mixed findings prompted the initiation of larger primary care studies, one of which has been published recently, the GAD-P study.[17] Unlike the primary care studies reviewed above, all of which were based on either DSM-III-R or ICD-10 diagnostic criteria for GAD, the GAD-P study was based on the more specific DSM-IV criteria. Building on a large nationally representative sample of 558 primary care doctors and DSM-IV criteria for GAD, GAD-P included a total of 20,245 unselected patients (age range 18–90) who visited their doctor on a target day in autumn 2000. Two particularly noteworthy strengths of the study are: (a) that all primary care attenders, irrespective of their reason for visiting the doctor's surgery, were included, allowing an estimation of the point prevalence of GAD and depression and their comorbid presentation in addition to an evaluation of associated impairment and disability; and (b) that all patients filled out a self-report diagnostic instrument and were independently evaluated by their doctors to examine recognition rates and diagnostic habits of clinicians. The data collected in GAD-P are very helpful in clarifying whether the prevalence of 'pure' GAD (no comorbid depression) among primary care attenders is really as low as suggested by some previous investigators.

With regard to point prevalence, the GAD-P study confirmed the results of previous primary care studies in showing that DSM-IV GAD is a very frequent disorder in primary care, with 5.3% (males 4.1%, females 6.2%) of patients meeting DSM-IV criteria for GAD. The prevalence of DSM-IV major depression, in comparison, was 4.4% (males 3.5%, females 5.0%). The study also revealed that an additional 20% of patients had at least some symptoms of generalized anxiety and/or depression, but failed to meet full diagnostic criteria for either disorder.

Unlike some previous studies discussed earlier Table 2.1 shows that among all GAD-P patients meeting GAD criteria, the majority did not have current major depression. The prevalences of pure GAD and comorbid GAD were 3.8% and 1.6%, respectively. This relatively high proportion of pure GAD is in agreement with the large primary care study of Ormel et al.,[12] which was based on ICD-10 criteria, but the finding differs from most of the previous studies that used DSM-III-R criteria and found that GAD in primary care is more likely to be comorbid than pure. A close inspection of the GAD-P data suggests that the high proportion of pure cases is the result of DSM-IV changes in the criteria list for GAD, in which many of the symptoms that could overlap with major depression were omitted. This change seems to have reduced the 'artificial' comorbidity found in earlier studies that was due to the less precise diagnostic criteria in the DSM-III and DSM-III-R systems.

The impairment measures used in the GAD-P study show that the majority of patients with pure GAD (66.7%) report having been impaired or completely disabled (unable to work) for at least one day in the past month because of their symptoms. This proportion was similar to that found for pure

Table 2.1 Point prevalence of pure and comorbid DSM-IV GAD in primary care (n = 17739 patients)

	Total		Males (n=7274)		Females (n=10465)	
	n	%	n	%	n	%
Neither generalized anxiety disorder nor major depression	16023	90.3	6725	92.5	9298	88.9
Pure generalized anxiety disorder	666	3.8	205	2.8	461	4.4
Pure major depression	772	4.4	251	3.5	521	5.0
Comorbid generalized anxiety disorder (with major depression)	278	1.6	93	1.3	185	1.8

Diagnoses are based on the DSM-IV algorithms for GAD and MDE according to the patient questionnaire. Only 17,773 out of the total of 20,245 subjects assessed fulfilled inclusion criteria and had a complete data set, including doctors' appraisal.

depression (68.4%), but significantly lower than for cases meeting criteria for both disorders (comorbid GAD: 81.1%). Interestingly, pure GAD, pure depression, and comorbid cases all reveal a significantly elevated risk to have impairment days due to somatic reasons, which seems to suggest important associations with somatic health for both conditions.[12] If impaired, the mean number of impairment/disability days among pure GAD cases was 9.9 days (mean ratio in comparison to non-GAD/depression cases: 1.4; 95% CI: 1.3–1.5), 15.3 days for pure depression (MR: 2.2; 95% CI: 2.1–2.4) and 16.5 days for comorbid GAD (MR: 2.3; 95% CI: 2.1–2.5).

The significant odds ratios in Table 2.2 also reveal that patients with pure and comorbid GAD and those with depression were high utilizers of health-care resources as compared to patients who did not have either condition. High utilization findings – controlled for physical morbidity – referred to primary care visits and specialist visits as well as consultation

of psychiatrists and psychologists. It is noteworthy, though, that only 19.8% of the pure GAD cases, 22.0% of the current major depression cases, and 20.8% of the comorbid group were currently in treatment for their condition. This low proportion of mental health treatment for both depression and GAD is remarkable, especially if one considers the fact that 38.9–42.4% of the patients indicated having received some form of treatment in the past because of their GAD or depression. This might be an indication of fairly poor doctor recognition of both anxiety and depression in primary care, even in cases with a past history of treatment for these conditions.

Another important measure of the burden of GAD is reflected in the comparatively high rates of suicidality: 25.4% of the GAD-P with pure GAD, 59.7% of those with pure depression, and 64.0% of those with comorbid GAD/depression reported having had frequent suicide thoughts over the past 4 weeks. These are much higher rates than those found among

Table 2.2 Impairment and disability measures in pure and comorbid GAD and major depression

	No GAD/ no DEP	Pure GAD		Comorbid GAD		Pure major depression	
	%	%	OR (95%CI)	%	OR (95%CI)	%	OR (95%CI)
Disabilities							
– disabled because of somatic problems	23.8	47.3	2.9 (2.4–3.4)	57.1	4.3 (3.3–5.7)	51.4	3.4 (2.9–4.0)
– disabled because of psychiatric problems	16.9	66.7	9.9 (8.3–11.7)	81.1	20.9 (14.8–29.0)	68.4	10.6 (8.9–12.7)
Treatment seeking							
–4+ primary care visits in the past 12 months	56.2	67.8	1.6 (1.4–2.0)	73.0	2.1 (1.6–2.8)	69.0	1.7 (1.4–2.1)
– 2+ visits to other specialist doctors	33.1	41.8	1.5 (1.2–1.7)	42.9	1.5 (1.2–2.0)	35.9	1.1 (1.0–1.3)
– psychiatrist	5.4	18.6	4.0 (3.2–5.0)	25.3	6.0 (4.4–8.1)	21.4	4.8 (3.8–6.1)
– psychotherapist	4.3	18.4	5.0 (3.9–6.3)	27.9	8.5 (6.4–11.4)	17.9	4.8 (3.8–6.1)
Suicidality/depr. episodes							
– frequent suicidal thoughts	6.3	25.4	4.8 (4.0–5.7)	64.0	26.3 (20.5–333.8)	59.7	21.9 (18.6–25.8)
– at least 2 depr. episodes	0.3	3.6	12.7 (7.5–21.4)	31.3	148.5 (100.2–220.0)	25.9	114.0 (79.6–163.3)
Therapy anxiety/depr.							
– never	78.7	41.4	ref.	29.9	ref.	36.8	ref.
– past	17.6	38.9	4.2 (3.5–5.0)	39.5	5.9 (4.4–7.9)	42.4	5.1 (4.4–6.0)
– current	3.7	19.8	10.2 (8.1–12.9)	22.0	21.2 (15.8–30.5)	20.8	12.1 (9.8–15.1)

Diagnoses are based on the DSM-IV algorithms for GAD and MDE according to the patient questionnaire. Except for the category 'Therapy for anxiety/depression' all Odds ratios are calculated controlling for age and gender using subjects with neither GAD nor depression as the reference. In contrast Odds ratios for Therapy used the category of never as the reference group.

primary care patients who meet criteria for neither GAD nor depression. Even in the case of pure GAD, where the rate of suicidality is lower than for depression or GAD/depression, the relative-odds compared to other primary care attenders is substantial (OR 4.8; 95% CI: 4.0–5.7). This effect of pure GAD on suicidality has rarely been highlighted in the previous literature.

The GAD-P study is currently awaiting replication in a number of Scandinavian countries (Finland, Sweden, Denmark,

Norway). If the findings of GAD-P outlined here are replicated in these other surveys, this will signal the need to dramatically shift our attention to the high proportion of GAD sufferers in primary care settings and even more to reducing the tremendous degree of burden associated.

Community studies

A comparison of the relative impairments associated with DSM-III-R GAD and major depression was performed by a recent study investigating jointly two US nationally representative samples.[18] The authors concluded that the impairments associated with DSM-III-R GAD are substantial and equivalent in magnitude to impairments associated with major depression, even after adjusting for other comorbid disorders.[18] Additionally, it was found that both pure GAD and pure major depression were associated with high levels of social role and work impairment. Highest levels of impairment were reported by respondents with comorbid GAD and major depression, a finding consistent with a number of studies reporting highest disability in subjects with multiple disorders.[12,16]

Evidence of GAD-specific impairments in the absence of major depression using the stricter DSM-IV criteria for GAD in a sample of the German population has also become available recently.[19,20] The focus of this study was on the disease-specific effects of pure GAD, pure major depression, and comorbid presentation of GAD and major depression on the number of days impaired in the past month, overall activity reduction in the past month, and self-perceived state of health. In addition, mean quality of life scores from all scales of the Short Form-36 Health Survey are reported for respondents with GAD and/or major depression.

As part of the German National Health Interview and Examination Survey—Mental Health Supplement (GHS), a nationwide, epidemiological study of mental health in Germany,[21] a random sample of over 4,000 subjects from the general population were personally interviewed by clinicians using the DSM-IV version of the Composite International Diagnostic Interview (CIDI). This study thus clarifies whether DSM-III-R findings for GAD can also be replicated in DSM-IV. To assess 'past month's days lost', respondents were asked how many days in the last four weeks they were completely unable to work or to carry out normal, everyday activities because of the syndrome. To assess 'past month's days limited', respondents were asked how many days in the last four weeks they were limited in their ability to carry out normal, everyday activities. Responses to these two questions were summed to result in the number of 'past month's days impaired'. Responses to these two questions were also used to calculate a past month overall work productivity reduction percentile, similar to the Reilly Work Productivity and Impairment questionnaire (WPAI).[22]

In addition, standard questions related to self-perceived impairment were included in the self-report packet completed by respondents. Respondents were asked if they perceived their state of health to be excellent, very good, good, fair, or poor. The German version of the Medical Outcomes Study Short Form-36 Health Survey (SF-36),[23,24] a quality of life measure that assesses health functioning and well-being across several domains, was also included in the self-report packet. This scale measures a broad range of health concepts (in eight domains) that are neither disease- nor treatment-specific. A score between 0 and 100 is given for each of the eight domains, and two summary scores can be calculated. For the eight specific domains, SF-36 standardized scale scores of 50–70 are usually regarded as indicating moderately reduced quality of life, whereas scores below 50 indicate a markedly reduced quality of life. The summary scale scores are designed to have a mean score of 50 and a standard deviation of 10 in a representative sample of the US population. The scale meets the psychometric standards of validity and reliability.[25–27]

Starting with impairment/disability days, Table 2.3 presents the outcomes of the impairment measures for the following mutually exclusive groups of respondents in this survey,

Table 2.3 Impairment measures for 12-month generalized anxiety disorder (GAD) and major depressive disorder (MDD) in the community (national sample, N=4181). Adapted from Wittchen et al.[20]

Impairment measure	Pure GAD[1] n=33			Pure MDD[2] n=344			GAD and MDD n=40			Neither GAD nor MDD n=3764		
	n	%w	95% CI	n	%w	95% CI	n	%w	95% CI	n	%w	95% CI
Self-perceived health												
Excellent or very good	3	10.1	3.1–27.9	34	12.4	8.7–17.3	0	0.0	– –	792	23.5	21.9–25.1
Good	14	43.1	26.4–61.5	202	56.2	50.2–62.0	20	48.6	32.4–65.2	2343	62.9	61.1–64.7
Fair or poor	16	46.9	29.6–64.9	108	31.5	26.2–37.2	19	51.4	34.9–67.6	571	13.6	12.5–14.8
Past month's days lost												
0	29	87.0	69.4–95.2	324	94.6	91.4–96.7	34	85.1	69.7–93.4	3731	99.3	99.0–99.5
1 or 2	1	2.1	0.3–13.4	2	0.4	0.1–1.7	0	0.0	– –	20	0.5	0.3–0.8
3 or more	3	10.9	3.6–29.0	18	5.0	3.0–8.1	6	14.9	6.6–30.3	13	0.2	0.1–0.4
Past month's days limited												
0	16	49.5	31.9–67.3	232	69.3	63.6–74.4	17	44.6	28.9–61.4	3473	93.6	92.7–94.3
1 or 2	0	0.0	– –	16	4.3	2.6–7.2	3	6.3	2.0–18.4	115	2.6	2.1–3.2
3 or more	17	50.5	32.7–68.1	96	26.4	21.6–31.9	20	49.1	33.0–65.4	176	3.9	3.3–4.5
Past month's days impaired (total)												
0	15	47.5	30.1–65.5	228	68.5	62.8–73.7	16	42.2	26.8–59.2	3463	93.3	92.5–94.1
1–2	1	2.1	0.3–13.4	17	4.4	2.6–7.2	3	6.3	2.0–18.4	120	2.7	2.1–3.2
3–5	4	16.2	6.2–36.3	24	6.4	4.2–9.7	2	3.9	1.0–14.5	95	2.2	1.7–2.7
6 or more	13	34.3	19.6–52.7	75	20.8	16.4–26.0	19	47.6	31.7–64.1	86	1.9	1.5–2.3
Past month's overall reduction in work productivity												
0	15	47.5	30.1–65.5	228	68.5	62.8–73.7	16	42.2	26.8–59.2	3463	93.3	92.5–94.1
0–10%	5	18.3	7.6–37.8	40	10.4	7.5–14.3	5	10.2	4.2–22.9	212	4.7	4.1–5.5
10–20%	4	5.5	2.0–14.5	16	4.2	2.5–7.1	6	13.7	6.2–27.8	37	0.8	0.6–1.2
20–30%	3	9.9	2.9–28.4	15	5.2	2.9–9.1	1	2.8	0.4–17.4	22	0.5	0.3–0.8
30–50%	3	7.9	2.5–22.7	16	3.9	2.3–6.5	2	8.0	2.0–27.3	11	0.3	0.1–0.5
>=50%	3	10.9	3.6–29.0	29	7.9	5.2–11.7	10	23.2	12.1–39.8	19	0.4	0.2–0.6

[1]Pure GAD contains those respondents with a 12-month GAD diagnosis and no 12-month MDD diagnosis. Respondents may have other DSM-IV disorders.
[2]Pure MDD contains those respondents with a 12-month MDD diagnosis and no 12-month GAD diagnosis. Respondents may have other DSM-IV disorders.

based on 12-month diagnoses: pure GAD (GAD without MDD), pure MDD (MDD without GAD), GAD and MDD, and neither GAD nor MDD. In this sample, greater impairments were reported by respondents with either or both disorders as compared to the impairments reported by respondents with neither of these disorders. Across all measures, respondents with comorbid GAD/MDD have the highest impairments, and the pure GAD respondents report slightly more impairments than the pure MDD respondents. Specifically, 23.2% of those with both GAD and MDD reported a reduction of at least 50% in their activities in the past month, compared to 10.9% of those with pure GAD and 7.9% of those with pure MDD. Concerning days impaired in the past month (a sum of days completely lost and days where the respondent was limited in the ability to carry out activi-

ties), 47.6% of the respondents with comorbid GAD/MDD had at least six days that were impaired, as compared to 34.3% of the pure GAD respondents and 20.8% of the pure MDD respondents.

For all of the quality of life subscales (Table 2.4), mean scores were significantly lower (indicating lower quality of life) in each of the GAD and MDD groups as compared to the group 'neither GAD nor MDD'. For the subscales general health, mental health, role limitations due to emotional health, and vitality, mean scores were significantly lower in the pure GAD group than in the pure MDD group. For the subscales general health, mental health, social functioning, and vitality, mean scores were significantly lower in the GAD and MDD group than in the pure MDD group. Physical summary score means in all three of the GAD and/or MDD groups were

Table 2.4 Quality of life associated with 12-month generalized anxiety disorder (GAD) and major depressive disorder (MDD)[1]. Adapted from Wittchen et al.[20]

SF-36 factors scale	Pure GAD n=33		Pure MDD n=344		GAD and MDD n=40		Neither GAD nor MDD n=3764	
	Mean	95% CI	Mean	95% CI	Mean	95% CI	Mean	95% CI
General health	46.58*≠	38.9–54.3	59.10*^	57.0–61.2	46.99*	40.8–53.2	68.39	67.8–69.0
Physical functioning	74.22*	64.6–83.8	82.96*	80.7–85.2	76.96*	69.2–84.7	88.37	87.7–89.0
Role physical	65.86*	51.5–80.2	72.23*	67.8–76.7	60.72*	45.3–76.1	85.48	84.4–86.5
Bodily pain	52.70*	43.6–61.8	56.33*	53.3–59.4	49.51*	41.8–57.2	69.07	68.2–70.0
Mental health	44.80*≠	39.7–49.9	56.60*^	54.5–58.7	42.93*	38.2–47.7	74.00	73.5–74.5
Social functioning	57.73*	48.3–67.1	70.12*^	67.1–73.1	57.10*	49.3–64.9	88.27	87.7–88.9
Role emotional	48.04*≠	35.8–60.3	67.98*	63.3–72.6	55.11*	40.0–70.2	91.48	90.7–92.3
Vitality	34.44*≠	29.1–39.8	46.95*^	44.8–49.1	36.21*	31.4–41.0	61.29	60.7–61.9
Physical summary[2]	46.40	42.2–50.6	47.49	46.4–48.5	45.20	41.2–49.2	49.38	49.1–49.7
Mental summary[2]	33.64*≠	30.7–36.6	41.55*^	40.2–42.9	35.11*	31.4–38.8	51.48	51.2–51.7

[1]Some scores contain missing data. All scores, except the sum scores, are standardized to 0–100; higher scores indicate better health.
[2]The sum scores are z-transformed using a standardized US population.
*Mean is significantly different from the mean in the 'neither GAD nor MDD' group; p<0.05.
≠Mean is significantly different from the mean in the 'pure MDD' group; p<0.05.
^Mean is significantly different from the mean in the 'GAD and MDD' group; p<0.05.

similar to the physical summary score mean in the 'neither GAD nor MDD' group. However, the mental summary score means were significantly lower for the pure GAD, pure MDD, and comorbid GAD/MDD groups, indicating lower quality of life in this general domain.

To show the extent to which GAD and MDD are each associated with increased impairments, odds ratios (ORs) from logistic regressions are presented in Table 2.5. These presented associations were controlled for age, gender, and the other mental disorders listed in the methods section. These results show that across nearly all of the outcome measures, pure GAD, pure MDD, and comorbid GAD/MDD are associated with significantly elevated impairments. The likelihood of perceiving one's health as fair or poor was significantly increased among respondents with pure GAD, pure MDD, and comorbid GAD/MDD as compared to respondents with neither disorder. In addition, the table shows that both disorders are significantly associated with having at least

six days in the past month when there is some disability to carry out everyday activities. Similarly, there was a significantly higher probability that respondents with either or both of these disorders would have a past month's activity reduction of at least 30%, as compared to respondents with neither of the disorders. Respondents with pure GAD, pure MDD, and comorbid GAD/MDD had significantly elevated odds for receiving an SF-36 mental summary score of 40 or below; however, respondents with GAD and/or MDD did not have significantly elevated odds for a physical summary score of 40 or below. No evidence was found for significant differences between any of the associations for pure GAD, pure MDD, and comorbid GAD/MDD.

As MDD is an episodic disorder that requires a minimum of two weeks of symptoms to receive a diagnosis, it is likely that some of the respondents with a 12-month MDD diagnosis were in complete remission at the time of the study interview, artificially

Table 2.5 Conditional associations of impairment measures of pure generalized anxiety disorder (GAD) and their comorbid presentation[1]

Measure of impairment	Pure GAD[2] n=33		Pure MDD[3] n=344		GAD and MDD n=40	
	OR	95% CI	OR	95% CI	OR	95% CI
Perceived health: fair or poor	4.38*	1.93–9.97	2.63*	1.93–3.59	2.69*	1.19–6.08
Past month's days lost: 3 or more	19.76*	3.84–101.62	12.82*	5.10–32.25	26.24*	6.72–102.37
Past month's days limited: 3 or more	14.13*	6.02–33.15	6.27*	4.39–8.95	11.68*	4.97–27.46
Past month's days impaired: 6 or more	13.87*	5.14–37.40	9.52*	6.19–14.65	21.05*	8.92–49.66
Overall activity reduction: >=30%	20.48*	6.62–63.40	15.99*	8.83–28.94	30.90*	11.81–80.86
SF-36 Physical summary score: <=40[4]	1.15	0.39–3.35	0.78	0.51–1.18	0.67	0.20–2.21
SF-36 Mental summary score: <=40[4]	22.33*	4.03–123.77	4.18*	2.86–6.12	5.95*	2.25–15.78

[1]OR=odds ratio; comparison group: no 12-month GAD and no 12-month MDD. Controlled for age, gender, and other psychopathology.
[2]Pure GAD contains those respondents with a 12-month GAD diagnosis and no 12-month MDD diagnosis.
[3]Pure MDD contains those respondents with a 12-month MDD diagnosis and no 12-month GAD diagnosis.
[4]<=40 is worse than approximately 84% of a representative US population.
*p<0.05; two-tailed z test.

lowering the severity of the impairment outcomes for MDD. Additional analyses were consequently performed to examine if greater associations with high impairment would be found for respondents with pure *current* MDD, and by respondents with *current* MDD comorbid with 12-month GAD (comparison group for all analyses: neither 12-month GAD nor 12-month MDD). These analyses resulted in high associations between MDD only and all the outcome categories: perceived health as fair or poor (OR=3.69, 95% CI: 2.34–5.80), at least six days impaired (OR=24.97, 95% CI: 14.67–42.50), at least 30% past-month activity reduction (OR=32.51, 95% CI: 16.59–63.70), and mental summary score <=40 (OR=5.99, 95% CI: 3.28–10.91). It is notable that none of these associations with impairment found for current MDD were significantly different from the associations reported for 12-month GAD. Respondents with current MDD comorbid with GAD had high associations with impairment. Particularly high odds were found for current MDD comorbid with GAD respondents to report at least six days impaired in the past month (OR=47.09, 95% CI: 17.13–129.41). Evidence was not found to show that these associations with impairment in comorbid cases were significantly different from the associations found for pure GAD and pure MDD, although for the outcome 'at least six days impaired in the past month' the difference between the associations for pure GAD versus current MDD comorbid with GAD approached significance (p=.073).

Convergent evidence for GAD-specific impairment from primary care and community studies

The main findings of GAD-P are in accordance with those of previous studies that have investigated the frequency and type of disabilities associated with DSM-III-R GAD in either representative primary care or in general population samples.[12,13,17,18] Given that GAD-P is the first community study to examine such issues by applying the stricter DSM-IV criteria for GAD on a large, nationally representative sample, the results add further to the credibility and reproducibility of the finding that GAD is associated with high impairment.

The GAD-P data also support the view that DSM-IV GAD is frequently comorbid with major depression, yet, using 12-month DSM-IV criteria there is evidence across studies that there is a considerable portion of pure GAD patients as well, namely about 40% in the community; for primary care only cross-sectional data are available to date suggesting that actually pure GAD is more frequent than comorbid GAD.

The disability experienced by people with GAD is thus not merely due to comorbid depression. This is clear not only from GAD-P, but from all the studies reviewed above. These studies confirm that GAD in itself, with or without comorbid depression, is a highly impairing clinical condition that results in significant and remarkable disabilities in terms of work productivity reductions, days where one is limited or even completely unable to perform everyday activities, and reductions in quality of life and well-being. Corresponding to the findings of Kessler et al.,[18] the elevated odds for GAD respondents to report high impairment were significant even when controlling for age, gender, and a wide range of other mental disorders. Interestingly, though, the German community study was unable to demonstrate that GAD is more impairing when it is comorbid with depression. One explanation for this could be that some of the respondents in the comorbid group were in partial or full remission of their depression at the time of the study interview. Supplementary analyses which restricted the comorbid cases to only those respondents with current depression and GAD suggest that current depression comorbid with GAD may be more strongly associated with high impairment than GAD in the absence of depression. It should also be mentioned that the proportion of respondents reporting high impairment on some of the measures (i.e., 'six or more' past month's days impaired, and '>=50%' past month's overall activity reduction) appears to be higher for the comorbid GAD/MDD respondents than for the pure GAD respondents.

Another remarkable finding of the studies is that the degree of impairment in each of the domains examined is impressively comparable between GAD and major depressive disorder not comorbid with GAD. While Schonfeld et al.[13] reported that major depression results in more reductions than GAD on most of the SF-36 scales, other studies found that the mean scores for GAD respondents were even lower than the mean scores for major depression on the scales assessing general health, mental health, role limitations due to emotional problems, and vitality. Wittchen et al.[17] and the study of Schonfeld et al.[13] both reveal that the domain of functioning affected most negatively by GAD and major depression is 'role limitations due to emotional problems'.

Not included in previous community studies is the documentation of disability associated with DSM-IV GAD and major depression in terms of specific amounts of reductions in work productivity, based on the Reilly Work Productivity and Impairment questionnaire (WPAI).[22] More than 50% of the respondents with GAD and no major depression and more than 30% of those with major depression and no GAD reported some reduction in their past month's activity.

Particularly remarkable, however, is the result that 23% of the respondents with comorbid GAD and major depression experienced reductions of at least 50% in their past month's activities.

An interesting and much broader comparative analysis of the impairment associated with GAD relative to other chronic conditions was carried out by Kessler et al.[28] in a study of the work-productivity losses associated with a wide range of chronic physical and mental disorders. This study was based on the MacArthur Foundation's recently completed Midlife Development in the US Survey (MIDUS),[28] a nationally representative survey of more than 3,000 people aged 25 to 74 years. This survey included a chronic conditions checklist that assessed the 12-month prevalence of the 20 most common chronic physical health problems reported in the US National Health Interview Survey in addition to five mental and substance-use disorders (i.e., major depression, panic attacks, alcohol dependence, GAD, and drug dependence). Also collected were data on the frequency of sickness absence days (i.e., missing an entire day of work because of ill health) and work cutback days (i.e., missing part of a day of work or a substantial cutback of productivity because of ill health) in the 30 days before the interview. The analysis consisted of evaluating the effects of the chronic conditions separately and together in predicting work impairment days (i.e., a weighted combination of sickness absence days and work cutback days). Adjusted mean levels were reported for selected physical conditions and for the five mental and substance-use disorders. Ulcers were associated with the highest average (i.e., mean) per capita impairment of any of the chronic physical conditions assessed in MIDUS: 5.8 d/mo. The other physical conditions for comparative purposes – arthritis, hypertension, asthma, and diabetes – were associated with average impairments of 3.1 to 3.5 days. GAD was not only associated with the highest average impairment of any of the mental or substance disorders (6.0 days), but, strikingly, people with GAD had the highest overall impairment of any of the more than two dozen disorders assessed in the survey. Also, consistent with the commonsense expectation that persistent worry would adversely influence 'knowledge work' more than manual labor, further analysis of these data found that the negative effect of GAD is most pronounced for college-educated people.

Patterns of treatment seeking

It was already noted above (see Table 2.2) that people with GAD are high utilizers of healthcare resources. Additional indirect evidence comes from the comparison of the relatively low 12-month prevalence rates of 2–3% for DSM-IV GAD found in the community with the considerably higher point prevalence rates of over 5% in primary care. The high prevalence of GAD in primary care ranks GAD together with MDD as the most frequent mental disorder seen in primary care. The significantly elevated number of visits to virtually all types of services supports the notion that GAD patients are high utilizers. This high proportion of patients with GAD, along with the vagueness of the patients' complaints, their chronic course and the primary care doctors' obvious deficits in dealing with such patients, has been reported to be an extremely burdening factor for doctors.[29] Further support comes from the previously mentioned NCS data that reveal that GAD and even more so comorbidity is a powerful predictor of help seeking among people with GAD.[5]

This finding of high health care utilization among people with GAD raises the important question of why so few people with GAD receive GAD-specific treatments. One plausible explanation is that GAD develops in some cases early in life associated with considerable comorbid pictures that hide the 'true' primary disorder. Another possibility is that GAD might have such an insidious onset that people affected try for a long time to cope without professional help. Yet a third, related, possibility is that many people with GAD might not realize that they have a serious mental disorder until secondary disorders develop. Another important consideration that almost certainly contributes to the low rates of treatment of GAD is that primary care doctors are unaware of effective screening and diagnostic tools and of effective modern treatments.

Although there are at this point no sufficiently detailed studies available to adjudicate definitively among these different interpretations, there is some scattered evidence for at least some core factors. Beesdo et al.[29] and Hoyer et al.[30] both demonstrated in their analyses that the vast majority of both patients and doctors do not know reliably what GAD actually is. Instead, and irrespective of the true comorbidity, GAD is frequently labelled as depression. Also, Hoyer pointed out that although more than two thirds of all DSM-IV GAD patients are correctly identified as clinically significant cases with a mental disorder, only 34.4% were correctly identified as having GAD. This very low positive recognition rate compares very unfavorably to the rates of correct diagnoses of depression of 64% in the abovementioned GAD-P.

These findings underline the fact that there is a clear need for primary care training and public awareness campaigns. These findings also lend some indirect support to the view that doctor and patient variables are key candidates for explaining the low numbers of patients receiving specific GAD treatment, whether appropriate or not.

Olfson et al.[31] have contributed evidence about delayed help-seeking patterns. They documented that speed of initial treatment contact after first onset of GAD is inversely related to age of onset of the disorder in general-population samples in the United States and Ontario, Canada. Approximately one third of people with GAD seek treatment in the year of onset of the disorder, whereas the average delay in initial treatment contact is more than a decade among people who delay beyond the first year. This is true not only in the United States, where there are financial barriers to seeking mental-health treatment, but also in Ontario, where such barriers are substantially fewer, arguing against the notion that financial barriers to treatment are an important determinant of treatment delays. Age at onset most likely is associated with speed of help seeking (Table 2.6) because of an increased recognition of anxiety as being problematic with increasing age of onset. The especially strong age-of-onset effect for seeking treatment in the year of onset is consistent with the findings of Hoehn-Saric et al.,[32] who found that most people with early-onset GAD report an insidious onset, whereas people with later-onset GAD are more likely to report an acute onset associated with a precipitating stressful event.

These pervasive delays in help seeking are of concern because there are effective psychological[33] and pharmacologic[3] therapies for GAD. Perhaps more worrying is that only a few people with GAD seek treatment even though most of them frequently seek primary care.

GAD is the most common anxiety disorder diagnosed in the primary care setting in the

Table 2.6 The effects of age at onset on speed of first treatment contact for generalized anxiety disorder in the United States and Ontario, Canada

| Age at onset (years) | Odds ratios* for treatment contact | | | |
| | In the year of onset of GAD | | In subsequent years | |
	U.S.	Ontario	U.S.	Ontario
<=12	1.0	1.0	1.0	1.0
13–19	22.5	7.5	1.4	1.3
20–29	73.6	35.8	2.0	2.0
>30	92.5	21.2	5.6	2.3

*These odds ratios were obtained by exponentiating logistic regression coefficients (in the model to predict contact in the year of onset of GAD), and by discrete-time survival coefficients (in the model to predict contact in subsequent years) from a model that included controls for cohort (in both) and time since onset (in the model to predict contact in subsequent years). There were 368 cases of GAD in the US sample and 153 in the Ontario sample.
GAD = generalized anxiety disorder.

United States[34] and many other parts of the world[35] because people with GAD commonly present with minor physical problems. Their anxiety is seldom treated, however, because primary care patients with GAD rarely include anxiety among their presenting complaints and primary care physicians often fail to recognize anxiety unless it is a presenting complaint.[36] This lack of recognition of the underlying psychological problem leads to frustration on the part of patients, who typically are not relieved of the secondary psychophysiologic symptoms that are usually their presenting complaints.[37,38] Patient screening and demand-management initiatives are being evaluated in an effort to increase recognition and treatment of GAD among these patients.

Another source of considerable concern regarding treatment of GAD is that research shows that many patients receive inadequate treatment. In a follow-up of the HARP sample, Goisman et al.[39] found that, as of 1996, dynamic psychotherapy was the most commonly used type of 'talk therapy' for patients with GAD. They found that only a few patients receive cognitive-behavioral therapy, even though treatment trials have documented the effectiveness of cognitive-behavioral therapy for GAD, whereas no such data exist for psychodynamic therapy. In a parallel analysis of the HARP data, Salzman et al.[40] found that as many as one third of patients seeking medical treatment for GAD in 1996 were unmedicated at interview. An unspecified additional proportion was under-medicated. Consistent with these results were the findings of Wang et al.,[41] who analyzed data from a large US telephone and mail survey conducted in 1996–97 and found that most patients in therapy for anxiety or mood disorders during those years received treatment that did not meet the minimum standards for effectiveness stipulated in treatment guidelines (i.e., certain AHCPR and APA guidelines).

Conclusion

The results reviewed in this chapter show convincingly that GAD, whether comorbid or pure, is an extremely distressing, impairing and disabling long-term illness, poorly recognized and treated. Perhaps because of the low rates of diagnostic recognition in the healthcare system and subsequently low uptake of GAD-specific treatments for the patients, we have to classify GAD patients as high utilizers of health-care resources with substantial cost implications, which adds to the considerable burden on the patient and his social network and work performance.

Further, these data are consistent with the position that GAD should be conceptualized as an independent disorder. Given the different prevalence rates for GAD and major depressive disorder, the different patterns of diagnostic overlap, and the differences in risk factors and associated features,[5,18] there seems to be little evidence that GAD is better conceptualized as a prodrome, a residual, or simply a severity marker of depressive disorders from this perspective.

Acknowledgements

The preparation of this paper was partially supported by the Global Research on Anxiety and Depression Network (GRAD), www.gradnetwork.com, through an unrestricted educational grant made possible by Wyeth-Ayerst Pharamaceutical and by grants O1EH9701/8 (National Morbidity Survey; PI: Dr Wittchen, Bundesministerium für Bildung, Forschung und Wissenschaft), W0129 (Generalised Anxiety and Depression in Primary Care; PI. Dr Wittchen, Wyeth Pharma, Münster) and U01-MH60220 (PI. Dr Kessler).

References

1. Maier W, Gaensicke M, Freyberger HJ, Linz M, Heun R, Lecrubier Y, Generalized anxiety disorder (ICD-10) in primary care from a cross-cultural perspective: a valid diagnostic entity?, *Acta Psychiatr Scand* (2000) 101:29–36.
2. Roy-Byrne P, Katon W, Broadhead WE, et al., Subsyndromal ('mixed') anxiety-depression in primary care, *J Gen Intern Med* (1994) 9:507–12.

3. Hackett D, Desmet A, Salinas EO, Venlafaxine XR in the treatment of anxiety, *Acta Psychiatr Scand* (2000) **102**(Suppl. 406):30–5.

4. Silverstone PH, Ravindran A, for the Venlafaxine XR 360 Canadian Study Group, Once-daily venlafaxine extended release (XR) compared with fluoxetine in outpatients with depression and anxiety, *J Clin Psychiatry* (1999) **60**:22–8.

5. Wittchen H-U, Zhao S, Kessler R, Eaton WW, DSM-III-R generalized anxiety disorder in the National Comorbidity Survey, *Arch Gen Psychiatry* (1994) **51**:355–64.

6. Kessler RC, Keller MB, Wittchen H-U, The epidemiology of generalized anxiety disorder, *Psychiatr Clin North Am* (2001) **24**:19–39.

7. Brown TA, Barlow DH, Liebowitz MR, The empirical basis of generalized anxiety disorder, *Am J Psychiatry* (1994) **151**:1272–80.

8. DiNardo P, Moras K, Barlow DH, Rapee RM, Brown TA, Reliability of DSM-III-R anxiety disorder categories: using the Anxiety Disorders Interview Schedule—Revised (ADIS-R), *Arch Gen Psychiatry* (1993) **50**:251–6.

9. Massion AO, Warshaw MG, Keller MB, Quality of life and psychiatric morbidity in panic disorder and generalized anxiety disorder, *Am J Psychiatry* (1993) **150**:600–7.

10. Sanderson WC, Barlow DH, A description of patients diagnosed with DSM-III-R generalized anxiety disorder, *J Nerv Ment Dis* (1990) **178**:588–91.

11. Kessler RC, The epidemiology of pure and comorbid generalized anxiety disorder: a review and evaluation of recent research, *Acta Psychiatr Scand* (2000) **102** (Suppl. 406):7–13.

12. Ormel J, Von Korff M, Ustun B, Pini S, Korten A, Oldehinkel T, Common mental disorders and disability across cultures: results from the WHO collaborative study on psychological problems in general health care, *JAMA* (1994) **272**:1741–8.

13. Schonfeld WH, Verboncoeur CJ, Fifer SK, Lipschutz RC, Lubeck DP, Buesching DP, The functioning and well-being of patients with unrecognized anxiety disorders and major depressive disorder, *J Affect Disord* (1997) **43**:105–19.

14. Stewart AL, Hays RD, Ware JE Jr., The MOS short-form general health survey: Reliability and validity in a patient population, *Med Care* (1988) **26**:724–35.

15. Spitzer RL, Kroenke K, Linzer M, et al., Health-related quality of life in primary care patients with mental disorders, *JAMA* (1995) **274**:1511–7.

16. Olfson M, Fireman B, Weissman MM, et al., Mental disorders and disability among patients in a primary care group practice, *Am J Psychiatry* (1997) **154**:1734–40.

17. Wittchen H-U, et al., GAD-P-Studie. Bundesweite Studie 'Generalisierte Angst und Depression im primaeraerztlichen Bereich', *Fortschritte der Medizin* (2001) **119** (Sonderheft 1):1–49.

18. Kessler RC, DuPont RL, Berglund P, Wittchen H-U, Impairment in pure and comorbid generalized anxiety disorder and major depression at 12 months in two National Surveys, *Am J Psychiatry* (1999) **156** (12):1663–78.

19. Carter RM, Wittchen HU, Pfister H, Kessler RC, One-year prevalence of subthreshold and threshold DSM-IV generalized anxiety disorder in a nationally representative sample, *Depress Anxiety* (2001) **13**;78–88.

20. Wittchen HU, Carter R, Pfister H, Montgomery SA, Kessler RC, Disabilities and quality of life in pure and comorbid generalized anxiety disorder and major depression in a national survey, *Int Clin Psychopharmacol* (2000) **15**;319–28.

21. Wittchen H-U, Mueller N, Storz S, Psychische Stoerungen: Haufigkeit, psychosoziale Beeintraechtigungen und Zusammenhaenge mit koerperlichen Erkrankungen, *Das Gesundheitswesen* (1998) **60**, (Sonderheft 2):95–100.

22. Reilly MC, Zbrozek AS, Dukes EM, The validity and reproducibility of a work productivity and impairment instrument, *Pharmacoeconomics* (1993) **4**:353–65.

23. Bullinger M, Kirchberger I, Ware J, The German SF-36 health survey. Translation and psychometric testing of a generic instrument for the assessment of health-related quality of life, unpublished.

24. Ware JE, Sherbourne CD, The MOS 36-item short form health survey (SF-36). I. Conceptual framework and item selection, *Med Care* (1992) **30**:473–83.

25. Brazier JE, Harper R, Jones NM, O'Cathain A, Thomas KJ, Userwood T, Westlake L, Validating the SF-36 health survey questionnaire: new outcome measure for primary care, *B M J* (1992) **305**:160–4.

26. McHorney CA, Ware JE, Raczek AE, The MOS 36-item short form health survey (SF-36): II. Psychometric and clinical tests of validity in

measuring physical and mental health constructs, *Med Care* (1993) **31**:247–63.

27. McHorney CA, Ware JE, Rogers W, Raczek AE, Lu JF, The validity and relative precision of MOS short- and long-form health status scales and Dartmouth COOP charts. Results from the medical outcomes study, *Med Care* (1992) **30** (Suppl 5):253–65.

28. Kessler RC, Mickelson KD, Barber V, et al., The effects of chronic medical conditions on work impairment. In Rossi AS (ed): *Caring and doing for others: Social responsibility in the domain of the family, work, and community*. (Chicago: University of Chicago Press 2001)

29. Beesdo K, Krause P, Höfler M, Wittchen H-U, Kennt der Allgemeinarzt die Generalisierte Angststoerung? Praevalenzschaetzungen, Einstellungen und Interventionen von Allgemeinaerzten vor Studienbeginn, *Muenchner Medizinische Wochenschrift – Fortschritte der Medizin 119. Jg. – Originalien, Sonderheft* (2001) 1:13–16.

30. Hoyer J, Krause P, Höfler M, Beesdo K, Wittchen H-U, Wann und wie gut erkennt der Hausarzt Generalisierte Angststoerungen und Depressionen? *Muenchner Medizinische Wochenschrift – Fortschritte der Medizin 119. Jg. – Originalien, Sonderheft* (2001) 1:26–35.

31. Olfson M, Kessler RC, Berglund PA, et al., Psychiatric disorder onset and first treatment contact in the United States and Ontario, *Am J Psychiatry* (1998) **155**:1415–22.

32. Hoehn-Saric R, Hazlett RL, McLeod DR, Generalized anxiety disorder with early and late onset of anxiety symptoms, *Compr Psychiatry* (1993) **34**:291–8.

33. Barlow DH, *Anxiety and its Disorders*. (New York: Guilford Press, 1988)

34. Barrett JE, Oxman TE, Gerber PD, The prevalence of psychiatric disorders in primary care practice, *Arch Gen Psychiatry* (1988) **45**:1100–6.

35. Ustun TB, Sartorius N *Mental illness in general health care: An international study*. (Chichester, New York: John Wiley & Son, 1995)

36. Ormel J, Van den Brink W, Koeter MW, et al. Recognition, management and outcome of psychological disorders in primary care: A naturalistic follow-up study, *Psychol Med* (1990) **20**:909–23.

37. Katon W, Von Korff M, Lin E, Lipscomb P, Russo J, Wagner E, Polk E, Distressed high utilizers of medical care: DSM-III-R diagnoses and treatment needs, *Gen Hosp Psychiatry* (1990) **12**:355–62.

38. Lin E, Katon W, Von Korff M, et al. Frustrating patients: Physician and patient perspectives among distressed high users of medical services, *J Gen Intern Med* (1991) **6**:241–6.

39. Goisman RM, Warshaw MG, Kelle MB, Psychosocial treatment prescriptions for generalized anxiety disorder, panic disorder, and social phobia, 1991–1996, *Am J Psychiatry* (1999) **156**:1819–21.

40. Salzman C, Goldenberg I, Bruce SE, Keller MB, Pharmacologic treatment of anxiety disorders in 1989 vs. 1996: Results from the Harvard/Brown Anxiety Disorders Research Program, *J Clin Psychiatry* (2001) **62**:149–52.

41. Wang PS, Berglund P, Kessler RC, Recent care of common mental disorders in the United States: Prevalence and conformance with evidence-based recommendations, *J Gen Intern Med* (2000) **15**:284–92.

3

Diagnosis and Evaluation of Generalized Anxiety Disorder Patients

Karl Rickels, Moira Rynn and Sarosh Khalid-Khan

Introduction

A comprehensive descriptive approach to the typology of anxiety disorders was first provided by Freud[1] more than 100 years ago. In 1894, Freud described a distinct syndrome, 'anxiety neurosis', which he separated from 'neurasthenia'. This work laid the foundation for the classification of anxiety disorders in a fashion that parallels Kraepelin's[2] role in the classification of schizophrenia and mood disorders.

Anxiety neurosis, according to Freud, consists of four major clinical syndromes: (1) general irritability, (2) chronic apprehension/anxious expectation, (3) anxiety attacks, and (4) secondary phobic avoidance.[1] Freud believed that anxious expectation represented the 'nuclear' symptom of anxiety neurosis. Two examples of 'anxious expectation' reported by Freud are (1) a woman who imagines that her husband will die each time he gives her a phone call and (2) the patient who finds two people standing in front of her house on returning home and automatically imagines that something has happened to her children. Freud provided the first description of *excessive worry* under the term *anxious expectation* because the worry is not constantly present but rather is present only in some circumstances. Apprehension, according to Freud, may be present chronically or 'come into consciousness suddenly, causing anxiety attacks' (now called *panic attacks*). These attacks can occur alone or may be associated with thoughts of sudden death.

Freud described anxiety symptoms as being primarily somatic ones that may occur either in a 'free-floating anxiety' or 'apprehension' state or in a 'sudden anxiety attack'. Freud suggested that the symptoms most likely to occur in anxiety states or anxiety attacks are trepidation, arrhythmia, dyspnea, sweating, nausea, heavy feeling in stomach, tremor, increased urination, increased appetite, diarrhea, vertigo, paraesthesias, pavor nocturnus, increased sensitivity to pain, decrease of sexual interest, and low self-esteem.

Freud also described two types of secondary phobic avoidance symptoms. He believed that chronic apprehension may lead primarily to simple phobias whereas vertigo and anxiety attacks may lead to agoraphobia. Also, he described anxious expectation as involving nervousness, apprehension, and free-floating anxiety. Finally, Freud already recognized in 1894 that anxiety neurosis commonly occurs in conjunction with other neuroses, a condition he called *mixed neurosis*. He observed that anxiety symptoms commonly occur in combination with those of neurasthenia, hysteria, and obsessions. Freud did not distinguish free-floating anxiety and chronic apprehension from anxiety attacks, but noted the existence of comorbid subthreshold anxiety.

The first edition of the Diagnostic and Statistical Manual for Mental Disorders[3] (DSM-I) was not published until 1952. The main impetus for developing the DSM-I were the changes that occurred in psychiatric thinking during and after World War II. Improved nomenclatures adopted by the armed forces and the Veterans Administration contributed significantly to the development of the DSM-I. Although psychoanalytic concepts were well known at the time, the experience of many soldiers with traumatic neuroses provided the final impetus for the acceptance of psychoanalysis into US psychiatry. Psychoanalysis emphasized the need to focus on non-psychotic, but presumably troubled, individuals. Psychoanalytic theory emphasized the psychological mechanisms that mediated between instinctual biological drives and pressures of the external environment.

The DSM-I,[3] and the DSM-II,[4] introduced in 1968, used the concept of neurosis as a major organizing principle in structuring the anxiety disorders. The predominant psychiatric theory in the United States at that time was that all psychopathology was secondary to anxiety, which, in turn, was caused by intrapsychic conflict. Psychosis was considered the result of such an excessive anxiety leaving

the ego crumbled and regressed, and neurosis was considered the result of a partially successful defense against anxiety that led to symptom formation.[5] In 1964, Rickels[6] described anxiety as:

. . . subjective feeling of heightened tension and diffused uneasiness, defined as the conscious and reportable experience of intense dread and foreboding, conceptualized as internally derived and unrelated to external threat. It is not merely fear because it lacks a specific object. It is a painful dread of situations, which symbolize unconscious conflicts and impulses. Anxiety can be partly bound by such mechanisms as phobias, obsessions and compulsions or it may be diverted into the soma, leading to somatization.

In the 1960s, psychiatrists realized that anxiety states were commonly comorbid with other anxiety states, at least at subthreshold levels, which led to severe impairment.

Anxiety disorders: from DSM-I to DSM-IV

A major change that occurred when psychiatric classifications shifted from DSM-I to DSM-II was the elimination of the term *reactions* applied to almost all diagnoses, including schizophrenia.[7] Meyer, never fond of Kraepelin's emphasis on classification, was most influential in believing that even psychotic disorders should be considered 'reactions' to environmental influences and stress.[8,9] During the late 1960s and early 1970s psychiatrists, especially those involved in clinical research, became disillusioned with the diagnostic system provided in DSM-I and -II. Many psychiatrists began to believe that one should move away from making a diagnosis based on unproven mechanisms, such as 'neurosis', and rather define psychiatric disorders in terms of age of onset, duration of illness, symptom patterns, and severity, irrespective of possible etiological underpinning. The Washington University group in St. Louis probably contributed most to this development in psychiatry and published a seminal article in 1972 entitled 'Diagnostic Criteria for Use in Psychiatric Research'.[10] The investigators defined 14 psychiatric disorders, including anxiety neurosis, obsessive-compulsive neurosis, phobic neurosis and hysteria. In the anxiety disorders, *free-floating anxiety* and *anxiety attacks* were still grouped under one diagnosis: *anxiety neurosis*.

Shortly afterwards, based on the Washington criteria,[10] the Research Diagnostic Criteria (RDC) were developed, which separated generalized anxiety disorder (GAD) from panic disorder.[11] GAD was defined as non-psychotic, generalized anxiety associated with persistent anxious mood of at least two weeks' duration, without frequent panic attacks, and with at least one secondary symptom (e.g., sleep difficulties, autonomic symptoms, muscle tension, tremor, worrying, or restlessness) and accompanied by impaired social functioning. This development led to the publication of the DSM-III by the American Psychiatric Association in 1980.[12,13]

The creators of the DSM-III believed strongly that the profession's advancement required a classification system that was atheoretic, with criteria that would be reliable and could provide the basis for testable hypotheses. This system should not be based on unproven etiological assumptions. Their intellectual roots were in St. Louis, not Vienna, and their intellectual inspiration was derived from Kraepelin, not Freud.[14,15]

Anxiety disorders in DSM-I were recorded under *psychoneurotic disorders* (i.e. reactions) and

in DSM-II under *neuroses*. However, with the advent of the DSM-III, neurosis became only a secondary qualifier. Thus, in DSM-III, the anxiety disorders had still in parentheses the notation 'or anxiety neurosis'. This continued with the DSM-III-R, published in 1987, in which the anxiety disorders had in parentheses, 'or anxiety and phobic neurosis'.[16] Finally with DSM-IV[17] these notations regarding neurosis were omitted.

Another major change that occurred from DSM-II to DSM-III was the removal from the *anxiety neuroses* (now called *disorders*) the hysterical, hypochondriacal, neurasthenic, and depressive neuroses, to be reclassified into somatoform, dissociative, and depressive disorders, separate from the anxiety disorders.[13] *Obsessive-compulsive neurosis* was renamed *obsessive-compulsive disorder*, and, for the first time, *post-traumatic stress disorder* and *atypical anxiety disorder* appeared as additional anxiety diagnoses. Atypical anxiety disorder became anxiety NOS (not otherwise specified) in the DSM-III-R and DSM-IV.

Generalized anxiety disorder (GAD)

The diagnostic term *generalized anxiety disorder* first appeared in DSM-III. However, generalized, persistent, and free-floating anxiety had already been described by Freud in 1894.[1] Anxiety neurosis, which in DSM-II included patients suffering from generalized symptoms of anxiety as well as those suffering from panic symptoms, now was separated into panic disorder and GAD, described by Freud as 'chronic apprehension/anxious expectation'. A duration criterion of one month was added to the GAD diagnostic criteria. Also, in the DSM-III, disorders first categorized in the DSM-II under *phobic neurosis* were now divided into *agoraphobia with panic attacks*, *agoraphobia without panic attacks*, *social phobia*, and *simple phobia*.

Even in DSM-I and DSM-II phobic neurosis was never included under anxiety neurosis but was always considered as separate from anxiety neurosis. In DSM-III the term GAD included all non-phobic anxiety patients with the exception of non-agoraphobic patients with frequent anxiety attacks (panic disorder). Interestingly, the organizers of the first wave of the Epidemiologic Catchment Area (ECA) national survey did not include GAD as a possible diagnosis in their research diagnostic interview,[18] clearly indicating the bias in the USA that the GAD diagnosis was only a residual diagnostic category. This bias was later disproven.[19] In fact one may argue that in many respects GAD can be considered the 'basic anxiety disorder' because its defining features, anxious expectation and hyperarousal, reflect the basic processes of anxiety. Unlike the other anxiety disorders, it has no clear behavioral marker to facilitate its differentiation and it is this fact that reduces inter-rater reliability.[20]

Clinical presentation

GAD is characterized by both psychological and physical symptoms. The psychological symptoms that dominate its presentation are a persistent feeling of fearful anticipation, repetitive worrying thoughts, irritability, poor concentration, and a feeling of restlessness. While the repetitive worrying thoughts tend to be of everyday matters, they can also be focused on physical symptoms.

The physical symptoms stem from two principal sources, muscle tension and autonomic hyperarousal. Muscle tension may cause tremor and muscle aches particularly in the back and shoulders. In addition it can cause tension headaches. Autonomic hyperarousal can affect every body system, causing numerous associated somatic symptoms, such as a feeling of tightness in the chest, overbreathing, palpitations, and chest pain. Not infrequently it is the physical symptoms of anxiety that are the presenting complaint, especially in general practice, leading patients to seek medical rather than psychiatric help. As a result, GAD patients frequently present in specialist medical clinics with unexplained physical symptoms. For example, a high proportion of patients with non-coronary chest pain have GAD.[21,22,23]

Generalized anxiety disorder in children

In the DSM-III-R, there were three anxiety disorders that could be diagnosed in children and adolescents: overanxious disorder, separation anxiety disorder, and avoidant disorder. Overanxious disorder (OAD) has been removed from the DSM-IV and children are now being diagnosed with generalized anxiety disorder. Both overanxious and generalized anxiety disorder share many features.[24] Avoidant behavior is now included in social phobia.[25] Separation anxiety disorder is still listed in the section entitled 'Disorders Usually First Diagnosed in Infancy, Childhood and Adolescence'.[26] This diagnosis requires four weeks' duration of symptoms. GAD in children is now characterized by excessive anxiety and worry in a variety of areas that the child finds difficult to control.

Often, making the diagnosis of a specific childhood anxiety disorder in children and adolescents can be challenging given the various factors that affect young people, such as family dynamics, intelligence, and socioeconomic status. Moreover, over time a child's anxiety symptoms may continue to evolve into another disorder or an additional anxiety diagnosis. A recent school-based prevention trial by Dadds et al.[27] found that 54% of untreated children identified by self-report and/or teachers' ratings with features of, but no full threshold, anxiety, developed an anxiety disorder over the six months of the study's monitoring period. In addition, older anxiety disordered children report significantly higher levels of anxiety and depression than younger children with the same diagnosis, suggesting that symptoms may worsen over time.[28] Children with overanxious disorder are likely to have other anxiety disorders as well.[29] A recent prospective study by Last et al.[30] suggests that, over a three to four year follow-up phase, children with anxiety disorders appear to be more likely than controls to develop new psychiatric disorders, primarily new anxiety disorders.

Diagnostic criteria for generalized anxiety disorder

In DSM-I, anxiety is described as diffuse and not restricted to definite situations or objects. It is characterized by anxious expectation, commonly associated with somatic symptoms. In DSM-II, anxiety is defined as anxious overconcern extending to panic, commonly associated with somatic symptoms, which must be distinguished from normal apprehension or fear. These definitions of anxiety changed with the DSM-III to 'generalized, persistent anxiety of at least 1 month's duration'.

Table 3.1 summarizes the various criteria used for diagnosing GAD in DSM-III, DSM-III-R, DSM-IV and ICD-10.[31] The definition of anxiety changes from 'persistent anxiety' in the DSM-III to 'unrealistic/excessive anxiety and worry about two or more life circumstances' in DSM-III-R. In DSM-IV it evolves into 'exces-

sive anxiety and worry about a number of events or activities' and 'it is difficult to control'. Also, DSM-IV requires fewer physical symptoms than does the ICD-10 for a diagnosis of GAD.

In the DSM-III-R, apprehensive expectation or worry was elevated to a cardinal or stem symptom, required for the diagnosis of GAD, regardless of how many other anxiety symptoms are present. Also, the word 'unrealistic' was omitted in DSM-IV, while the worry became 'excessive' and 'difficult to control'. The criterion of duration of illness shifted from one month in the DSM-III to six months in the DSM-III-R and DSM-IV and to several months in ICD-10.

In the DSM-III, ancillary symptoms included an unspecified number of symptoms from 3 of 4 categories: (1) apprehensive expectation, (2) motor tension, (3) autonomic hyperactivity, and (4) vigilance. In DSM-III-R, these ancillary symptoms changed to 6 of 18 specified symptoms, eliminating the apprehensive expectations category, because this category had become a primary or cardinal criterion for the diagnosis, now defined as 'worry'. In DSM-IV, the ancillary symptoms were further reduced and involve only 3 of 6 symptoms, selected from the categories of motor tension and vigilance, omitting the autonomic category. In children, only one ancillary symptom is necessary. This shift in symptom focus, away from somatic symptoms to those of psychological concern, and a change in duration from one to six months, may have profound consequences for conceptualization of the disorder and its treatment.

Many anxious patients treated in the family practice setting present themselves with somatic rather than psychological symptoms. In an epidemiologic study, Bridget et al.[32] compared primary care patients described as 'somatizers' (n = 47), those patients who focus on somatic symptoms and who endorse

Table 3.1 Shift in criteria to diagnose generalized anxiety disorder (GAD)

Criteria	DSM-III	DSM-III-R	DSM-IV	ICD-10
Anxiety	Persistent anxiety	Unrealistic/excessive anxiety and worry (apprehensive expectation) about 2 or more life circumstances	Excessive anxiety and worry (apprehensive expectation) about a number of events or activities; worry difficult to control (includes overanxious disorder of childhood)	Anxiety is generalized and persistent, free-floating, dominant symptoms are highly variable. A variety of worries or foreboding are frequently experienced
Duration	1 month	6 months	6 months	Several months
Ancillary symptoms	Unspecified number of symptoms from 3 of the 4 following categories • Apprehensive expectation • Motor tension • Autonomic • Vigilance	≥6 of 18 specified symptoms from the following 3 categories • Motor tension (n=4) • Autonomic (n=9) • Vigilance (n=5)	≥3 of the following 6 symptoms • Restlessness/mental tension • Fatigue • Poor concentration • Irritability • Muscle tension • Sleep disturbance	Unspecified number of symptoms from 3 categories • Apprehension (worry about future, feeling 'on edge', difficulty concentrating) • Motor tension (restlessness, fidgeting, tension headaches, trembling, inability to relax) • Autonomic over-activity (lightheadedness, sweating, tachycardia, epigastric discomfort, dizziness, dry mouth, . . .)
Associated features	Mild depressive symptoms	Mild depressive symptoms	• Muscle tension • Somatic symptoms • Depressive symptoms • Exaggerated startle response	
Impairment in social and occupational functioning	Rarely more than mild	Rarely more than mild	Significant distress and impairment	
Exclusions	Not due to another mental disorder such as depression or schizophrenia	• Anxiety/worry, unrelated to another disorder (e.g. panic, psychosis) • Anxiety does not occur only during mood disorder or psychotic disorder • Anxiety not related to organic factors (e.g. hyperthyroidism, caffeine intoxication)	• Anxiety/worry not due to another anxiety disorder (e.g. panic, psychosis) • Anxiety does not occur exclusively during mood disorder or psychotic disorder • Anxiety not due to medical conditions such as hyperthyroidism or substance abuse	Must not meet full criteria for depressive episode, phobic disorder, panic disorder, obsessive-compulsive disorder

symptoms justifying a psychiatric DSM-III diagnosis only on extensive questioning, with patients described as 'psychologizers' (n = 55), that is, patients presenting with psychological symptoms. Because of a predominance of 'somatizers' in primary care, 'psychologizers' had to be oversampled. Both groups of patients were compared with patients with bona fide somatic complaints (n = 91). Somatizers and psychologizers were significantly more anxious than were the control group with somatic complaints only. Interestingly, more somatizers (58%) than psychologizers (33%) received a diagnosis of GAD, whereas the reverse was true for major depression (38% vs. 68%).

In the DSM-III and DSM-III-R associative features included 'mild depressive symptoms' whereas in the DSM-IV, in addition to unspecified severity of depressive symptoms, various somatic symptoms such as those of muscle tension were added. Finally, the definition of impairment, which in DSM-III and III-R was considered 'only mild', is considered in DSM-IV as 'producing clinically significant distress or impairment in social, occupational, or other important areas of function'.

The emphasis in DSM-III-R and DSM-IV is on worry, which is secondarily defined as 'apprehensive expectation'. The authors believe that apprehensive expectation would be a more relevant and useful term, a term which is not synonymous with worry. Finally, the exclusion criteria for all classifications include that the focus of anxiety or worry is not: (1) on symptoms of another disorder (e.g., panic disorder or social phobia), (2) part of a mood disorder or psychotic disorder, (3) related to substance abuse, or (4) related to organic causes (e.g. hyperthyroidism or caffeine intoxication).

The diagnostic criteria for GAD in the ICD-10, preferred by many European clinicians, prominently features 'anxiety which is generalized and persistent and not restricted to partic-

ular or environmental circumstances, i.e. it is free floating'.[31] The criterion of duration of symptoms is 'several months.' The dominant symptoms are described as 'highly variable', and are subsumed under the three headings of apprehension, motor tension, and autonomic activities. Complaints include consistent nervousness, trembling, muscle tension, lightheadedness, sweating, palpitations, dizziness, epigastric discomfort, fear, and worry.

Research diagnostic criteria were also developed for the ICD-10 (Diagnostic Criteria for Research-10).[33] They have increased the duration criterion from 'several months' to 'at least 6 months' and mandate that at least 4 of 22 specific symptoms be present for a diagnosis. These symptoms are classified as: (1) autonomic symptoms (n = 4), (2) symptoms of chest or abdomen (n = 4), (3) symptoms involving mental state (n = 4), (4) general symptoms (n = 6), and non-specific symptoms (n = 4). They are based on the DSM-III-R symptom list.

Because the ICD-10 provides slightly more relaxed diagnostic criteria than the DSM-IV classification system, it is probably clinically more realistic and meaningful, particularly for treatment decisions. Its definition of anxiety as generalized, persistent, and free-floating lacks the US psychiatry's excessive focus on worry while still mentioning 'apprehension' as one of several key symptoms of anxiety; it also has a less rigid duration criterion.

DSM-IV: worry focus, duration, severity

Based on many years of experience in diagnosing and treating patients with GAD, particularly in the family practice setting, the authors believe that severity of anxious psychological and somatic symptomatology, and not 'focus on worry' or 'duration,' is one of the most important criteria for the diagnosis of GAD. A similar finding was recently reported by Bienvenu et al.[34] Using Diagnostic Interview Schedule data from the 1993 follow-up study of the Baltimore cohort of the Epidemiologic Catchment Area program, subjects were classified into five mutually exclusive groups: (1) DSM-III-R GAD; (2) 6–month duration of worry or anxiety with 6 associative symptoms but not fulfilling excessive worry criteria; (3) 1–month duration of anxiety with 6 associated symptoms; (4) 1-month duration of anxiety with less than 6 associated symptoms; and (5) no anxiety. The results indicated that subjects in the first three groups were homogeneous with regard to demographics and comorbidity profiles, but, that their profiles differed significantly from those of the other two groups. Thus, the requirement of 6 of 18 symptoms (DSM-III-R), most likely representing more symptom severity without worry as a cardinal symptom or longer duration, produced groups with a particular epidemiological profile and elevated *general anxiety* from a commonly subthreshold to a clear diagnostic category. These data call into question the utility of the DSM-IV diagnostic construct. The most important differentiation between 'ill' and 'not ill' groups was the presence of at least 6 associated symptoms, not worry or duration. Further evidence that the number of symptoms present may be important to the validity of the diagnosis was provided in a twin study by Kendler et al.[35]

Further relevant publications include the following. Rogers et al[36] subclassified GAD as primary or secondary and observed that patients with primary GAD were more likely to be in an anxious episode at intake and less likely to have a secondary diagnosis of agoraphobia, social phobias, simple phobia, posttraumatic stress disorder, alcohol abuse or drug abuse disorder, or major depression

disorder. But both GAD groups were similar in terms of prevalence and treatment outcome, an observation relevant for treatment. Olfson et al.[37] found in family practice sites more subthreshold patients with GAD (6.6%) than full-threshold patients with GAD (3.7%), further supporting the need to reassess present diagnostic GAD criteria. This is particularly true if one considers that *subthreshold* does not necessarily translate into 'less ill', but only that *some* GAD criteria, such as 6 months' duration or excessive worry, were not fulfilled. Subthreshold patients were still significantly more socially impaired than were controls. Similar conclusions were drawn by Marcus et al.[38] using data from the National Medical Expenditures Survey.

DeBeurs et al.[39] reported on vulnerability factors for experiencing a state of anxiety in an elderly population. Anxiety symptoms were assessed with the Hospital Anxiety and Depression Scale-Anxiety Subscale[40] and not according to DSM-IV criteria. The investigators found neuroticism (i.e. trait anxiety) and female sex as the most likely predictors of chronic anxiety symptoms, with significant life events, primarily the death of one's partner, leading to acute anxiety. Thus, a high level of neuroticism, similar to Akiskal's 'anxious temperament'[41] may be considered a vulnerability factor for acute and chronic anxiety episodes, even if these episodes do not fulfil GAD criteria. Finally, Dugas et al.[42] present empirical evidence for a conceptual model of GAD that features as its key process variable 'intolerance of uncertainty', and which was pivotal in distinguishing subjects with GAD from normal controls. Three additional variables (i.e., 'beliefs about worry', 'poor problem orientation', and 'cognitive avoidance') further contributed to differentiation of the subject groups. Earlier, these investigators had shown that 'intolerance of uncertainty' also clinically discriminated women who met GAD criteria from women who did not.[43]

Thus, number and severity of anxiety symptoms, and possibly high intolerance of uncertainty, seem to be the most relevant diagnostic criteria for GAD, not duration of illness and not excessive worry focus. As part of a diagnostic assessment,[44] severity of anxiety symptoms may easily be measured with scales such as the Hamilton Anxiety Scale (HAM-A),[45] the Hopkins Symptom Checklist (HSCL),[46] the Hospital Anxiety and Depression Scale (HAD),[40] the General Health Questionnaire (GHQ)[47] or by a variety of other scales. Interestingly, simply an increase in the number of associated symptoms in DSM-IV necessary to make a diagnosis from 3 to 4 might well allow an increase of anxiety symptom severity.[48] Akiskal[41] proposes that many of the chronic worry symptoms of GAD might represent trait symptoms, or, as he describes them, 'anxious temperament', on which state anxiety symptoms are added at certain times, commonly as a response to chronic stress. Similarly, several years ago, Rickels and Schweizer[49] proposed the diagnostic term *double anxiety*, recognizing the chronic sustained underlying anxiety of many years' duration, which is probably a trait phenomenon, onto which the acute anxious episode has been added. It is this acute episode that is particularly responsive to psychopharmacological therapy,[50] while trait anxiety or temperament may possibly be more responsive to various psychotherapeutic approaches.

GAD *and other psychiatric disorders: some diagnostic considerations*

GAD can be clearly distinguished from panic disorder if a patient experiences frequent, spontaneous panic attacks and agoraphobic symptoms. Many patients with GAD, however, do have occasional limited anxiety/panic attacks (i.e. subthreshold). An even closer overlap probably exists between GAD and social phobia. While patients with clear-cut phobic avoidant behavior may be distinguished easily from patients with GAD, patients with social anxiety without clear-cut phobic avoidant behavior may overlap in symptoms with patients with GAD and differentiation may be difficult. In the authors' clinical experience such patients frequently have GAD as the primary disorder and social anxiety at subthreshold levels. The cardinal symptoms of GAD commonly overlap with those of social phobia, particularly if the social phobia is general and not focused on a specific phobic situation. For example, free-floating anxiety may cause the hands to perspire and may cause a person to be shy in dealing with people in public, and thus many patients with subthreshold social phobic symptoms should be given, in the authors' opinion, a diagnosis of GAD and not generalized social phobia. The distinctions between GAD and obsessive-compulsive disorder, acute stress disorder, and post-traumatic stress disorder are by definition not difficult. At times, however, it may be difficult to distinguish GAD from adjustment disorder with anxious mood or from anxiety not otherwise specified, particularly if the adjustment disorder occurs in a patient with high levels of neuroticism or trait anxiety or type C personality disorder. Table 3.2 presents some features distinguishing GAD from other psychiatric disorders.

Patients with lifetime comorbid diagnoses of other anxiety or depressive disorders, not present for 1 year or more and not necessitating treatment during that time period, meet a primary diagnosis of current GAD. Patients with concurrent threshold anxiety or mood

Table 3.2 Features distinguishing GAD from other disorders

Disorders	Features
Generalized Anxiety Disorder	Excessive anxiety, worry and apprehensive expectation, free-floating anxiety, many somatic complaints, no phobic avoidance behavior, no severe depressed mood or anhedonia. No frequent panic attacks.
Panic Disorder	Recurrent, self-limiting, unexpected anxiety (panic) attacks and anticipatory anxiety of another attack.
Social Phobia	Avoidance, not only fear of social or performance situations in a public setting.
Agoraphobia	Fear of being trapped in a situation (which can be non-social) where escape is difficult or embarrassing. Clearly avoidant phobic behavior.
Separation Anxiety (Children)	Fear of being separated from a parent or guardian, yet socially 'comfortable' at home.
Avoidant Personality Disorder (Cluster C)	Includes a more general inadequacy or awkwardness in a social context (patient may lack even simple social skills).
Adjustment Disorder with Anxiety	A response to a clear stress; once the stressor has terminated, duration of symptoms less than 6 months. Symptoms may be quite similar to those in GAD.
Major Depressive Disorder	Primary symptoms are severe depressed mood and marked anhedonia.
Post-traumatic Stress Disorder	A traumatic event is persistently re-experienced.
Specific Phobia	Unreasonable fear and avoidance of a specific object or situation.

disorders should be diagnosed according to those disorders and not as primary GAD.[51] Somatization disorders are classified separately from anxiety disorders in DSM-IV. Some of these, particularly undifferentiated somatization disorder, may overlap with GAD and be diagnostically difficult to distinguish. The authors believe that, as long as psychological symptoms of anxiety are present and predominant, patients should probably be given a primary diagnosis of GAD. Anxiety due to medical conditions, e.g. hyperthyroidism, and anxiety caused by medication, e.g. caffeine,

amphetamines, or drugs of abuse, must be excluded.

Suggestions to the evaluating physician

The two major shifts in DSM diagnostic criteria for GAD from DSM-III to DSM-IV have markedly redefined this disorder. One shift involves the duration criterion from 1 to 6 months, and the other, the increased emphasis on 'worry', as well as an emphasis on psychological, rather than somatic, symptoms. This decision has had the consequence of losing a large population of patients suffering from generalized anxiety that is more transient and somatic in its focus, and who typically present to primary care physicians, and probably receive most often the diagnosis of anxiety NOS or adjustment reaction. Clinicians may want to consider using the ICD-10 qualification of illness duration of 'several months' to replace the more rigid DSM-IV criterion of '6 months' and to move away from the DSM-IV focus on 'excessive worry' as the cardinal symptom of anxiety, focusing instead on 'free-floating anxiety.' Finally, the adjective 'excessive' should be omitted since it is not used in DSM-IV for the definition of other primary diagnostic criteria, such as depressed mood for major depressive disorder for example.

One may also want to consider the separation of trait (chronic) from state (acute) anxiety.[48,49] It is not yet known whether the presence of some personality characteristics, such as anxious personality, cluster C personality, anxious temperament, or increased neuroticism, are prerequisites for developing an anxiety disorder, or are only vulnerability factors that may predispose some patients to develop a full-blown anxiety disorder.[52]

Anxiety defined as 'non-psychotic *generalized* anxiety without phobic symptoms and without major depressions' seems to be a valid description of many anxious patients with threshold and subthreshold generalized anxiety symptoms in potential need of treatment by their family physician. Depending on duration of symptoms, treatment may be either short term or long term. This definition will allow doctors to diagnose and treat the many patients not fulfilling a GAD diagnosis under

Table 3.3 Anxiety conceptualization	
Type of anxiety	**DSM-IV diagnoses**
Acute anxiety • Transient anxiety (acute reactions to situational stress) • Short-term anxiety (reaction to specific life events)	• Non-pathological reaction to stress • Acute stress disorder • Adjustment disorder • Anxiety NOS
Subacute anxiety • Minor anxiety • Brief anxiety • Brief, intermittent anxiety	• Adjustment disorder • Anxiety NOS
Chronic anxiety • Continuous anxiety • Intermittent anxiety	• GAD • Anxiety NOS
Double anxiety • Mild to moderate continuous anxiety with episodic bouts of full-fledged anxiety	• GAD • Anxiety NOS

DSM-IV rules or who are presently diagnosed as anxiety NOS or adjustment disorder. Anxious patients frequently present not with anxious worry but with physical complaints to their primary care physician. They are also frequent users of health-care services. Table 3.3 suggests an anxiety conceptualization that would be helpful for the family physician in diagnosing and treating his/her patients.[50]

Treatment by the family physician could be provided on a gradient of severity and illness duration, ranging from the passage of time and psychosocial support by the family physician, to prn and short-term benzodiazepine therapy, to various psychosocial or chronic pharmacological treatments with such medications as buspirone, antidepressants, and occasionally, in selected circumstances, also benzodiazepines.

Similar to dysthymic disorder, which has only recently been demonstrated to be a highly impairing depressive illness,[53,54] even if not fulfilling DSM-IV major depressive disorder severity criteria, subthreshold generalized anxiety disorder is similarly reported to cause great discomfort and high impairment in functioning.[37,38]

GAD, as defined by DSM-IV, has become a rather reliable diagnosis, but because of its many restrictions it has questionable validity. Similar concern about the validity of many DSM-IV diagnoses was recently expressed by McHugh,[55] who pointed out that the DSM-IV allows one to identify over 2000 subcategories of depression. McHugh believes that the commitment to improved reliability in the DSM-IV has too long deferred the issue of validity.

In conclusion the authors hope that in future DSM revisions, diagnostic splitters, so influential in the past, will be joined by diagnostic lumpers, to ensure a more balanced approach to psychiatric diagnoses, considering not only reliability but also validity.[55,56]

References

1. Freud S, The justification for detaching from neurasthenia a particular syndrome: the anxiety neurosis. Collected papers, Vol. 1. London, Hogarth Press, 1953. Originally published in 1894

2. Kraepelin E, Psychiatrie: Ein Lehrbuch fur Studierende und Aerzte, 5th edn. Leipzig, JA Barth, 1896

3. American Psychiatric Association, Diagnostic and Statistical Manual of Mental Disorders, (Washington, DC: American Psychiatric Association Mental Health Service, 1952)

4. American Psychiatric Association, Diagnostic and Statistical Manual of Mental Disorders 2nd edn. (Washington DC: American Psychiatric Association, 1968)

5. Klein DF, Anxiety reconceptualized. In Klein DF, Rabkin J (eds) Anxiety: New Research and Changing Concepts. (New York: Ravin Press 235:243–5, 1981)

6. Rickels K, The use of psychotherapy with drugs in the treatment of anxiety, Psychosomatics (1964) 5:111–5

7. Spitzer RL, Wilson PT, A guide to the American Psychiatric Association's new diagnostic nomenclature, Am J Psychiatry (1968) 124:41–51

8. Grob GN, Origins of DSM-I: A study in appearance and reality, Am J Psychiatry 1991 148:421–31

9. Meyer A, Letter to Southard EE, Dec 16, 1918, in Adolf Meyer Papers. Baltimore, Chesney Medical Archives, Johns Hopkins Medical Institutions.

10. Feighner JP, Robins E, Guze SB, Woodruff RA, Winokur G, Munoz R, Diagnostic criteria for use in psychiatric research, Arch Gen Psychiatry (1972) 124:57–63

11. Spitzer RL, Endicott J, Robins E, Research diagnostic criteria. Arch Gen Psychiatry (1978) 35:773–82

12. American Psychiatric Association, Diagnostic and Statistical Manual of Mental Disorders, 3rd edn.

(Washington, DC: American Psychiatric Association, 1980)

13. Spitzer R, Williams J, Skodol A, DSM-III: The major achievements and an overview, *Am J Psychiatry* (1980) 137:151–64

14. Kroll J, Philosophical foundations of French and US nosology, *Am J Psychiatry* (1979) 136:1135–8,

15. Bayer R, Spitzer R, Neurosis, psychodynamics, and DSM-III, *Arch Gen Psychiatry* (1985) 42:187–96

16. American Psychiatric Association, Diagnostic and Statistical Manual of Mental Disorders, 3rd edn. rev. (Washington, DC: American Psychiatric Association, 1987)

17. American Psychiatric Association, Diagnostic and Statistical Manual of Mental Disorders, 4th edn. (Washington, DC: American Psychiatric Association, 1994)

18. Robins LN, Regier DA, Psychiatric disorders in America: The epidemiologic catchment area study. (New York: The Free Press, London: Collier MacMillan Publishers, 1991)

19. Wittchen HU, Hoyer J, Generalized anxiety disorder: nature and course, *J Clin Psychiatry* (2001) 62 (Suppl 11):15–19

20. Brown TA, Barlow DH, Liebowitz MR, The empirical basis of generalized anxiety disorder, *Am J Psychiatry* (1994) 151:1272–80

21. Logue MB, Thomas AM, Barbee JG et al., Generalized anxiety disorder patients seek evaluation for cardiological symptoms at the same frequency as patients with panic disorder, *J Psychiatr Res* (1993) 27:55–9

22. Wulsin LR, Arnold ML, Hillard JR, Axis I disorders in E.R. patients with atypical chest pain, *Int J Psychiatry Med* (1991) 21:37–46

23. Kane FJ, Harper RG, Wittels E, Angina as a symptom of psychiatric illness, *South Med J* (1988) 81:1412–6

24. Kendall PC, Warman MJ, Anxiety disorders in youth: Diagnostic consistency across DSM-IIIR and DSM-IV, *J Anxiety Disord* (1996) 10:452–63

25. Kendall PC, Brady EU, Comorbidity in the anxiety disorders of childhood. In Craig KD & Dobson KS (eds) *Anxiety and depression in adults and children* (Newbury Park, CA: Sage Publications, 1995)

26. Tracey SA, Chorpita BF, Douban J, Barlow DH, Empirical evaluation of DSM-IV generalized anxiety disorder criteria in children and adolescents, *J Clin Child Psychiatry* (1997) 26:404–14

27. Dadds MR, Spence SH, Holland DE, Barrett PM, Laurens KR, Prevention and early intervention for anxiety disorder: A controlled trial, *J Consulting and Clin Psychiatry* (1997) 65 (Suppl 4):627–35

28. Strauss CC, Behavorial assessment and treatment of overanxious disorder in children and adolescents, *Behav Modif* (1988) 12:234–51

29. Last CG, Hersen M, Kazdin AE, Finkelstein R, Strauss CC, Comparison of DSM-III separation anxiety and overanxious disorders: Demographic characteristics and patterns of comorbidity, *J Am Acad of Child & Adolescent Psychiatry* (1987) 26:527–31

30. Last CG, Perrin S, Hersen M, Kazdin AE, A prospective study of childhood anxiety disorders, *J Am Acad of Child Adolesc Psychiatry* (1996) 35(Suppl 11):1502–10

31. World Health Organization, The ICD-10 Classification of Mental and Behavioural Disorders: Clinical Descriptions and Diagnostic Guidelines (Geneva, WHO, 1992)

32. Bridget K, Goldberg D, Evans B, Sharpe T, Determinants of somatization in primary care, *Psychol Med* (1991) 21:473–83

33. World Health Organization, The ICD-10 Classification of Mental and Behavioural Disorders: Diagnostic Criteria for Research (Geneva, WHO, 1993)

34. Bienvenu OJ, Nestadt G, Eaton WW, Characterizing generalized anxiety: Temporal and symptomatic thresholds, *J Nerv Ment Dis* (1998) 186:51–6

35. Kendler KS, Neale MC, Kessler RC et al., Clinical characteristics of familial generalized anxiety disorder, *Anxiety* (1994/1995) 1:186–91

36. Rogers MP, Warshaw MG, Goisman RM et al., Comparing primary and secondary generalized anxiety disorders in a long-term naturalistic study of anxiety disorders, *Depress Anxiety* (1999) 10:1–7

37. Olfson M, Broadhead WE, Weissman MM, Leon AC, Farber L, Hoven C, Kathol R, Subthreshold psychiatric symptoms in a primary care group practice, *Arch Gen Psychiatry* (1996) 53:880–6

38. Marcus SC, Olfson M, Pincus HA, Shear MK, Zarin DA, Self-reported anxiety, general medical conditions, and disability bed days, *Am J Psychiatry* (1997) 154:1766–8

39. DeBeurs E, Beekman ATF, Deeg DJH, Van Dyck R, Van Tilburg W, Predictors of change in anxiety symptoms of older persons: Results from the longitudinal aging study Amsterdam, *Psychol Med* (2000) 30:515–27

40. Zigmond AS, Snaith RP, The hospital anxiety and depression scale, *Acta Psychiatr Scand* (1983) 67:361–79

41. Akiskal HS, Toward a definition of generalized anxiety disorder as an anxious temperament type, *Acta Psychiatr Scand* (1998) 98 (Suppl 393):66–73

42. Dugas MJ, Gagnon F, Ladouceur R, Freeston MH, Generalized anxiety disorder: A preliminary test of a conceptual model, *Behav Res Ther* (1998) 36: 215–26

43. Freeston MH, Rheaume J, Letarte H, et al., Why do people worry? *Personality and Individual Differences* (1994) 17:791–802

44. Stein DJ, Seedat S, Niehaus DJH, Pienaar W, Emsley RA, Psychiatric algorithms for primary care, *Prim Psychiatry* (2000) 7:45–67

45. Hamilton M, The assessment of anxiety by rating, *Br J Med Psychol* (1959) 32:50–5

46. Derogatis LR, Lipman RS, Rickels K, Uhlenhuth EH, Covi L, The Hopkins Symptom Checklist (HSCL): A measure of primary symptom dimensions. In: *Psychological Measurements in Psychopharmacology*. Mod. Prob. Pharmcol-psychiatri. P Pichot (ed.) (Basel: Karger 1974 7:79–110)

47. Goldberg DP, Steele JJ, Johnson A, Smith C, Ability of primary care physicians to make accurate ratings of psychiatric symptoms, *Arch Gen Psychiatry* (1982) 39:829–33

48. Starcevic V, Bogojevic G, The concept of generalized anxiety disorder: Between the too narrow and too wide diagnostic criteria, *Psychopathology* (1999) 32:5–11

49. Rickels K, Schweizer E, Long-term treatment of anxiety disorders: Maintenance treatment studies in anxiety disorders: Some methodological notes, *Psychopharmacol Bull* (1995) 31:115–23

50. Rickels K, Schweizer E, The spectrum of generalised anxiety in clinical practice: The role of short-term, intermittent treatment, *Br J Psychiatry* (1998) 173 (Suppl 34):49–54

51. Sussman N, Toward an understanding of the symptomology and treatment of generalized anxiety disorder, *Primary Psychiatry* (1997) 4:68–81

52. Paris J, Anxious traits, anxious attachment, and anxious-cluster personality disorders, *Harvard Rev Psychiatry* (1998) 6:142–8

53. Pennix BW, Leveille S, Ferrucci L, van Eijk JT, Gurainik JM, Exploring the effect of depression on physical disability: longitudinal evidence from the established populations for epidemiologic studies of the elderly, *Am J Public Health* (1999) 89:1346–52

54. Wells KB, Stewart A, Hays RD, et al., The functioning and well-being of depressed patients: results from the Medical Outcomes Study, *JAMA* (1989) 262: 914–9

55. McHugh PR, Beyond DSM-IV: From appearances to essences, *Psychiatric Research Report* (2001) 17:2–15

56. Mack AH, Forman L, Brown R, Frances A, A brief history of psychiatric classification: From the ancients to DSM-IV, *History of Psychiatry* (1994) 17:515–23

4

Toward a Psychological Model of the Etiology of Generalized Anxiety Disorder

Susan Mineka, Iftah Yovel and Suzanne L Pineles

Generalized anxiety disorder (GAD) has sometimes been referred to as the 'basic anxiety disorder', suggesting that understanding the etiological and maintaining factors for GAD may help us better understand other anxiety disorders, and perhaps major depression as well.[1] In the search for etiological and maintaining factors in GAD psychologists in the past 15–20 years have focused their attention primarily on the cardinal characteristic of GAD – pathological worry. Thus the central focus of this chapter will be how the universal experience of worry becomes pathological. However, in attempting to shed light on this central issue, we will first review recent findings on the role of negative affectivity in GAD and discuss how such findings impact our understanding of the best way to conceptualize GAD diagnostically. Next we briefly discuss the role of cognitive biases toward threatening information in GAD and how these biases may play a role in the development of pathological worry. Then, we review recent findings on the positive and negative consequences of worry. Finally, we propose a model (drawing on the vicious circle behavior phenomenon studied in animals) that delineates a possible mechanism for the development of pathological worry.

Generalized anxiety disorder: conceptual and diagnostic issues

As discussed in more detail in other chapters in this volume, there has been some serious debate about how best to conceptualize GAD, including major questions about the validity of GAD as an independent Axis I disorder. Some researchers have argued that GAD is not an Axis I disorder but simply reflects an extreme personality trait that predisposes to other anxiety and mood disorders, while others have proposed that GAD is better conceptualized as a personality disorder (Axis II) rather than as an Axis I disorder. Yet others have maintained that GAD is best thought of as an Axis I disorder. In framing this debate, we will first consider the hierarchical symptom structure for GAD and related emotional disorders and how this may inform these issues regarding how best to conceptualize GAD from a theoretical and diagnostic standpoint.

GAD and negative affectivity

Numerous studies have shown high levels of comorbidity between GAD and major depression – both at a diagnostic and a symptom level (see Chapter 1). In addition, findings of behavior genetic studies suggest that these two disorders are genetically indistinguishable (i.e., the same genetic factors influence the risk for both disorders[2,3]). There is also evidence that the common genetic diathesis is best conceptualized as a personality trait commonly known as neuroticism or negative affectivity, which refers to a proneness to experience negative mood states.[3] Such findings regarding the comorbidity among the various emotional disorders have triggered the development of structural models such as Clark and Watson's tripartite model of anxiety and depression.[4] In these models, symptoms of anxiety and depression that tend to co-occur are grouped into broader factors, and the structure of the model represents the theoretical and empirical relationships among these factors. The highly influential tripartite model proposed that three different symptom factors underlie the symptomatology of major depression and the anxiety disorders.[4–6] The symptom factor known as negative affect or general distress, which parallels the broad personality dimension of negative affectivity or neuroticism, is the non-specific factor that is shared by all these syndromes. In other words, the symptoms that are grouped by this broad factor are frequently experienced by both anxious and depressed individuals. These

symptoms of negative affect often stem from a general tendency towards experiencing negative mood states – negative affectivity or neuroticism (e.g., sadness, anxiety, hostility, irritability, fear, and self-blame).[4–6]

In addition, according to the tripartite model both anxiety and depression are further defined by factors or groups of symptoms that are relatively specific to each type of disorder. Anhedonic depression (i.e., symptoms of low positive affect such as lack of energy and loss of interest and pleasure) is the specific factor associated with depression, while the anxious arousal factor (i.e., feelings of somatic tension and hyperarousal, including symptoms such as dizziness, shortness of breath, or dry mouth) was thought to be relatively unique to anxiety.[4] Later, however, Brown et al.[5] showed that the anxious arousal factor is not elevated for all anxiety disorders, but is relatively specific to panic disorder. Moreover, the model that showed the best fit to the data in the Brown et al.[5] study showed that, controlling for negative affect, the correlation between the factor that was defined by the GAD symptoms and the anxious arousal factor was significantly negative. This interesting result (discussed further later in this chapter) supports previous findings that GAD and worry are actually associated with autonomic inflexibility or the suppression of autonomic symptoms.[7] Indeed, the only factor that clearly differentiates between GAD and major depression is anhedonic depression, which is associated only with depression. The high comorbidity rates between GAD and major depression[3,4] are therefore explained in the tripartite model by the fact that both these syndromes are characterized by high levels of negative affect. In fact, in the Brown et al.[5] study GAD was the disorder that had the strongest association with this broad factor. Next we consider how structural models like the tripartite model may inform the debate about how best to conceptualize GAD.

GAD as a predisposition to other disorders?

The strong association that GAD has with the broad personality dimension of negative affectivity (NA) or neuroticism has led some researchers to suggest that GAD may be primarily a characterological predisposition to other emotional disorders rather than an Axis I disorder.[1] This notion would be consistent with known features of GAD, including its substantial comorbidity with other emotional disorders and its relatively early average age of onset.[8] Important support for this perspective also comes from findings that trait NA/neuroticism is a known risk factor common to most, if not all, anxiety and mood disorders.[9,10] Thus rather than being an Axis I disorder, some believe that GAD may better be conceptualized as the extreme end of a broad personality trait that serves as a general vulnerability to most emotional disorders.[11] However, even though in some cases the basic symptoms and traits associated with GAD may only serve as a predisposition to other disorders, it is also clear that for some people these symptoms become prominent enough to warrant a separate diagnosis of GAD.[11]

GAD as a personality disorder?

Another view is that GAD is best conceptualized as an Axis II and not as an Axis I disorder. According to DSM-IV, in order to be diagnosed as a personality disorder, the pattern of the personality traits needs to be inflexible, maladaptive, persistent, and pervasive across a wide range of situations, and cause significant distress or impairment in important areas of functioning. Undoubtedly, the basic features of GAD meet these criteria.

In addition, a personality disorder should be manifest in at least two different areas (cognition and negative affectivity for GAD). The only criterion for personality disorders that is questionable for GAD is that the pattern has to be stable and of long duration, with an onset that can be traced back to adolescence or at least to early adulthood. Indeed, studies have shown that in most cases GAD patients find it difficult to report a specific age of onset of the disorder or report an onset which dates back to childhood.[12] Others, however, report a later onset in a significant number of cases, which is often a response to some kind of a life stress.[13] As Brown[11] noted, it is possible that this bimodal distribution of the age of onset of GAD represents two separate etiological pathways to this disorder. Taking this perspective, only the first type of early-onset (but not later-onset) GAD may fit the current definition of a personality disorder.

In summary, according to the basic criteria of personality disorders in DSM-IV, most cases of GAD (those with early onset) might best be conceptualized as an Axis II rather than an Axis I disorder (although we are not aware of any formal proposals to do this). In any case, whether it is defined as an Axis I anxiety syndrome, an Axis II personality disorder, or merely as a predisposition to other emotional disorders, it is clear that GAD is strongly associated with high levels of negative affectivity. Later, we will try to show how this central feature of GAD may be important, but not sufficient, to understanding the etiology of this disorder.

Psychopathology of GAD

According to the DSM-IV, the most prominent feature of GAD is clinically distressing, excessive, pervasive, and uncontrollable worry about a number of events or activities (such as work, health, or school performance). These criteria were designed to differentiate pathological worry seen in GAD from the universal experience of everyday worry. This differentiation is based on features that are related to the worry process (e.g., frequency, perceived controllability), as well as on the effect the worry process has on the person's life, but not on the content of the worries, which is quite similar in nonclinical anxiety.[1,14] In addition, the focus of the worry in GAD should not be confined to themes or features of other Axis I disorders, such as being embarrassed in public (social phobia) or having a panic attack (panic disorder). This exclusion criterion is important because the process of worry is not unique to GAD, but its content is less circumscribed in GAD.[15]

Given that excessive and uncontrollable worry is the cardinal characteristic of GAD according to DSM-IV, can our understanding of the strong relationship between GAD and high negative affectivity help us understand why only a subset of people with high negative affectivity develop uncontrollable worry? Are there additional psychological processes needed to explain the development of uncontrollable worry? Many would agree that additional processes are necessary, in part simply because a structural descriptive level of analysis tells us little about the process of developing full-blown GAD.

Since generalized anxiety disorder emerged as a distinct diagnostic category over 20 years ago, significant advances have been made in understanding the psychopathological processes involved in this disorder. However, as will be seen, there are also some apparent paradoxes in the pattern of findings that have emerged which remain to be resolved at the theoretical level. For example, if everyone

worries to some degree, what leads some people to worry uncontrollably? If worry is experienced as an unpleasant activity, why would it be so terribly difficult for some people to control? Further, if worry has both positive and negative consequences, as research seems to show, why don't the negative consequences make it less rather than more likely to occur? Before we propose a potential mechanism for uncontrollable worry, let us start with some of the new and exciting findings of the past two decades on generalized anxiety and its central component – worry.

Anxiety and mood-congruent cognitive biases for threat

In the past two decades a great deal of research on mood and anxiety disorders has focused on mood-congruent *cognitive biases* for emotional material. Mood-congruent cognitive biases are said to occur when people display selective or non-veridical processing of emotion-relevant material.[16] The three primary kinds of bias are in attention, interpretation, and memory. For generalized anxiety the two most prominent kinds of cognitive bias are attentional and interpretive biases for threatening information. Given our limited cognitive resources, our information-processing systems must constantly make 'decisions', many of them unconscious and automatic, about which stimuli in the environment will be detected and processed and which will be ignored or discarded. Demonstration of mood-congruent *attentional biases* requires that the emotional meaning of stimuli (e.g., neutral, positive, or threatening) interacts with an individual's current mood state (e.g., neutral, positive, or anxious) to affect which stimuli are attended to. For example, when generally anxious (but not non-anxious) individuals read a newspaper they are likely to have their attention drawn to news stories with threatening content more than to those with neutral or positive content.[17,18]

Since about 1985 numerous studies (pioneered by Mathews and MacLeod and their co-workers[18,19]) using several different sophisticated information-processing paradigms have demonstrated that individuals with GAD (as well as other anxiety disorders) show automatic attentional biases toward threat cues when there is a mixture of threatening and non-threatening cues available in the environment – even when these cues are presented subliminally. The biases are said to be automatic or preconscious because they occur at such an early stage in the information-processing sequence that the anxious individual is not aware of, and has no volitional choice in, where his or her attention is directed, as occurs with subliminal stimuli.[18,19,20] Several (but not all) studies demonstrated that high trait anxious subjects also show such preconscious attentional biases.[17,18]

Several theorists and researchers have speculated that these attentional biases almost certainly play a role in maintaining the disorder once it has developed, and may play an etiological role as well. Specifically, if you're already anxious (either by virtue of having high trait anxiety or GAD) and your attention tends to be drawn automatically toward threatening stimuli in the environment, this is only going to serve to maintain or even exacerbate your anxiety. Consistent with this, several studies have shown that this kind of bias is usually no longer significant following successful treatment.[21,22] That such biases may serve as vulnerability factors, and hence play an etiological role as well, is now supported by at least three studies. In each study a measure of subliminal threat interference taken during a non-stressful baseline period was the best predictor of the amount of state anxiety and

distress experienced at a later point in time during or following a significant stressor.[17,23,24] Obtaining such similar results is particularly noteworthy because each of the three studies used the same cognitive vulnerability marker but different stressors and different types of subjects.

In addition to attending preferentially to threatening material, anxious individuals (relative to controls) estimate the likelihood of future negative events happening to them as higher. When asked, they also generate more numerous different negative (but not positive) future events that are going to happen to them than do controls.[25] Moreover, several studies have shown that anxious individuals are more prone to interpret ambiguous material in a threatening manner than are controls. For example, anxious individuals show biased interpretations when they hear ambiguous sentences (e.g., 'the doctor examined little Emma's growth' or 'they discussed the priest's convictions').[26] As with attentional biases, these *interpretive biases* can be seen as playing a role in maintaining generalized anxiety: if you are already anxious and find yourself automatically interpreting ambiguous situations in a negative manner, this should only serve to maintain or even exacerbate your anxiety. There is also now some preliminary evidence that interpretive biases may play an etiological role as well.[27]

The benefits and functions of worry.

As reviewed above, attentional and interpretive biases associated with generalized anxiety seem implicated both as risk factors and as playing a role in maintaining or exacerbating anxiety over time. Another independent line of research on worry – started by the pioneering work of Borkovec and colleagues – has also contributed significantly to understanding why GAD tends to be such a chronic disorder. As discussed later, worry seems to promote more worry and to maintain anxiety. This important line of investigation reveals a rather complex pattern of findings that can seem somewhat paradoxical. After reviewing this pattern of findings, we will propose a potential theoretical explanation of this apparent paradox.

Borkovec[28,29] and Wells,[30,31] among others, have investigated what people with GAD think the benefits of worrying are, as well as what functions the process of worry actually serves. In one study, people with GAD were asked what they believed were the most common *benefits* derived from worry. The five most common were: (1) superstitious avoidance of catastrophe; (2) actual avoidance of catastrophe by generating ways of preventing it; (3) avoidance of deeper emotional topics by distraction through worrying; (4) coping and preparation for the anticipated negative event; (5) motivating device to accomplish what needs to be done.[28,29,31] Believing or expecting that worry serves these functions may help account for why it can become a favored coping strategy for some.[28,32]

Moreover, new developments in understanding what *functions* worry actually serves have given new insights into why the worry process may be so self-sustaining. As discussed by Borkovec,[29] when people with GAD worry their emotional and physiological responses to aversive imagery are actually suppressed. Several studies have also shown that suppression of sympathetic activity occurs more generally (not just during aversive imagery) both in GAD and in non-clinical worry (see Chapter 8). Borkovec hypothesizes that this

suppression of emotional and aversive physiological responding serves to negatively reinforce[‡] (that is, increase the probability of) the worry process. He further hypothesizes that because worry seems to suppress physiological responding, it also serves to keep the person from fully experiencing or processing the topic that is being worried about – a necessary process if reduction (extinction) of that anxiety is to occur.[29,33] Thus the threatening meaning of the topic being worried about is maintained because full processing is prevented. For these and other reasons Borkovec et al. have postulated that worry serves as a *cognitive avoidance response*, which is negatively reinforced by the reduction in physiological and psychological emotional responses that ensues during and following worry. Cognitive avoidance occurs because behavioral avoidance of the distal and remote threats people so often worry about is not feasible.

Borkovec and colleagues also hypothesize that worry serves in an additional way as a conditioned cognitive avoidance response. As noted above, people believe that worry is an effective method of preventing future negative events. Although worry itself may in reality have no or very little impact on the occurrence or non-occurrence of such negative events, people who worry nevertheless are usually superstitiously reinforced for it because most of the things they worry about never occur (or if they occur are far less serious than anticipated). In one study of students,[34] both those with GAD and non-anxious controls were asked to keep diaries of every topic they worried about for at least two weeks, and also to record whether these things indeed happened. For the

---

[‡]Positive reinforcement occurs when a response leads to delivery of a positive reward (food, praise, money); the effect is an increase in the probability of that response in the future. Negative reinforcement occurs when a response leads to termination or avoidance of an aversive situation (such as working very hard to get through a huge pile of work or working very hard to avoid a reprimand at work); here again, the effect is an increase in the probability of that response in the future.

students with GAD, 85% of the topics they worried about turned out better than expected (70% for non-anxious controls). Thus, whether or not worry is actually involved in preventing expected bad outcomes, it is clearly superstitiously negatively reinforced as if it did most of the time.

In summary, there is considerable evidence at this point, mostly generated by Borkovec and colleagues, that both people with GAD and non-anxious controls often experience superstitious negative reinforcement (e.g., by the non-occurrence of bad outcomes) and real negative reinforcement (e.g., by the suppression of somatic sympathetic activity) for the worry process (see Figure 4.3). Moreover, both people with GAD and non-anxious controls also believe and expect that the worry process serves some important cognitive avoidance functions. Together, these two lines of evidence on worry as a negatively reinforced activity may help partially explain why worry becomes such a chronic mental activity for people with GAD. Indeed, Wells and Butler[35] further suggested that 'the immediate anxiety-reducing or anxiety-controlling properties of worry will lead to a loss of control of the activity as it is reinforced'. However, we believe that by themselves these negative reinforcement functions of worry cannot explain why the worry process in people with GAD has come to be perceived as an *uncontrollable activity* (a defining feature for DSM-IV). For example, people with GAD report having less control over their worrying and less success in reducing their worries as compared to non-anxious controls.[14] Yet most people do not generally lose control over reinforced activities (negatively or positively) including over worry itself – especially ones

that are somewhat unpleasant to begin with (e.g., being praised for having done a good job does not make most people workaholics, or taking the trash out to avoid smells of rotten food does not make people compulsive cleaners).[‡] For a more complete analysis of why worry has come to be perceived as uncontrollable in people with GAD, we believe one must also consider the negative consequences of worry.

The negative consequences of worry

As noted by Borkovec et al.[29] and Wells,[31] among others, the effects of worry are not all positive by any means. Phenomenologically worry itself has been described 'primarily as negative, verbal linguistic . . . activity'.[29] Thus, even though worry may serve in some ways as an effective escape or avoidance response, it is not a neutral activity but rather a negative one. In addition, worry may lead to a greater sense of danger and anxiety because of all the catastrophic outcomes generated (which can also serve as further trigger topics for more worry).[31] Moreover, although worry may serve an immediate dampening function for sympathetic arousal, it also seems to be associated with long-term maintenance of anxiety because extinction of the anxiety is prevented. In addition, people who worry about something negative subsequently tend to have more negative intrusive thoughts than occur in people who do not worry in the same situation. For example, Wells and Papageorgiou[36] had unselected individuals watch a gruesome film. Following the film some were told to relax, some were told to imagine the events in the film, and some were

---

[‡]The primary exception to this occurs with some stimulant addictive drugs that operate directly and powerfully on positive reinforcement pathways in our brains; some people obviously do lose control over such reinforcers.

told to worry in verbal form about the film. Over the next few days people in the worry condition reported experiencing the most intrusive images from the film. In this case one might say the worry process was punished by the occurrence of the negative intrusive images. (See also Butler et al.[37] for related results.) Based on findings such as these Wells and Butler[35] concluded 'Individuals who are prone to worry... perhaps to avoid images, are likely to engage in an activity that pollutes the stream of consciousness with an increasing frequency of intrusive thoughts.' Or, as noted above, in the language of learning theory, the process of worry can have punishing properties (as well as negatively reinforcing properties).

In addition to worry having potentially aversive and punishing effects, some evidence also shows that attempts to control thoughts and worry can have further pernicious effects by paradoxically leading to an increased experience of intrusive thoughts and enhanced perception of being unable to control them.[31,35] Although unfortunately none of the relevant studies are on people with GAD, the findings are of potential interest and importance for GAD nonetheless. In one relevant study Roemer and Borkovec[38] had unselected subjects either suppress or express their thoughts (for 5 minutes) about one of three kinds of situations they had personally experienced in the past: a depressing, an anxious, or a neutral situation. Then all subjects were told to express thoughts about the same situation for a second 5-minute period. Mood ratings were taken once before and once after these two tasks. Results showed that initial attempts to suppress anxious or depressing thoughts can later lead to their increase as well as to greater anxious and depressed mood (although see Purdon[39]). Related findings have also been reported by Wenzlaff et al.[40] for depressed (and undoubtedly also anxious)

students who showed a resurgence of unwanted negative thoughts after a period of suppressing such thoughts. Moreover, Salkovskis and Campbell[41] found that when participants were asked to suppress personally relevant intrusive thoughts, they showed more intrusive thoughts both during and after the suppression period than did a control group not asked to suppress such intrusive thoughts.

In summary, several different lines of research have shown that there are a number of negative aspects to, and consequences of, the worry process: 1) worry itself is experienced as a negative verbal linguistic activity; 2) worry can lead to a greater sense of danger because of all the catastrophic outcomes generated; 3) worry can lead to more worry and/or negative intrusive thoughts; 4) attempts to suppress worrisome negative thoughts or experiences may later lead to more of those thoughts and to more anxious and depressed mood than if the negative thoughts had been expressed in the first place. Given this pattern of findings in which the consequences of worry can be somewhat aversive and punishing, one might expect that the punishing consequences would lead to the extinction of worrying as a coping response because punishment is often an effective way of extinguishing responses. Thus, these aversive consequences of worry, when considered in conjunction with findings that the worry process may also serve a cognitive avoidant (negatively reinforcing) function, seem to leave us with somewhat of a puzzle. If the worry process is both negatively reinforced and punished, why do the negative reinforcement effects seem to predominate in those with GAD, who spend a large portion of each day worrying and who have a perception that their worry is uncontrollable? Some have referred to this as part of the 'neurotic paradox'[29] but a careful analysis of what the underlying mechanism may be that is producing it seems lacking.

Why does worry persist if it is both punished and reinforced?: A possible resolution of this apparent paradox

If worry can be seen to function, at least in part, as a cognitive avoidance response, then one potential resolution of this puzzle comes from considering the extensive literature on the consequences of punishing avoidance responses.[42] Although punishment of avoidance responses does sometimes lead to cessation of the avoidance responses, in many cases the opposite occurs, that is, punishment of avoidance responses can actually lead to *increases* in avoidance responding, which sometimes persists almost indefinitely. In a typical experiment on avoidance learning, animals (although the same basic effects have also been observed in humans) are presented with a discriminative stimulus (S^D) which is followed some seconds later by an aversive stimulus such as shock (setting the occasion for conditioning of fear to the S^D) (see Figure 4.1-early). First, the animal learns to make a designated response to escape the shock, but later they learn that if they respond quickly enough after the onset of the S^D they can reduce their fear (S^D turned off) and completely avoid the shock (avoidance response) (see Figure 4.1-late). Once the avoidance response (AR) is well established the experimenter can turn off the shock and the animal often keeps responding for prolonged periods whenever the S^D is presented, i.e., the animal shows pronounced resistance to extinction of the AR even though the response is no longer necessary to avoid the shock.[43,44] Although the mechanisms underlying this pronounced resistance to extinction of ARs was for decades the topic of serious debate,[43,45] one plausible theory that probably explains part of the effect is that fear

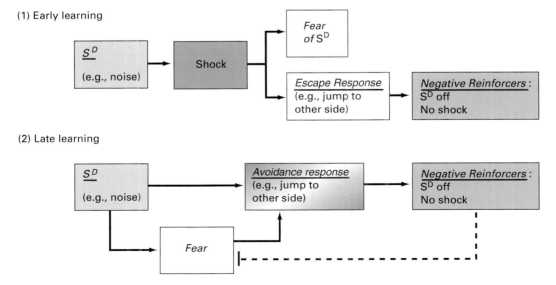

Figure 4.1 Early and late phases of avoidance learning. Note: Solid line with an arrow indicates one box leads to (or increases the likelihood of) the other. Dashed line with a bar indicates one box inhibits (or decreases the likelihood of) the other.

of the S^D motivates the AR, and that the response is negatively reinforced by fear reduction (see Figure 4.1-late).

Approximately 50 years ago theorists became interested in discovering ways to facilitate the extinction of avoidance responding once the response is no longer necessary to avoid shock. Several researchers discovered (in an attempt to facilitate extinction of such ARs) that delivering a short punishing shock whenever the animal makes the AR, often leads to paradoxical *increases* in responding! This phenomenon has been replicated many dozens of times across a wide variety of paradigms and several species. It has been labeled *vicious circle behavior* by some, and self-punitive behavior by others. There have been a variety of interpretations of vicious circle behavior.[42,46] However, the most prominent one hypothesizes that the punishing shocks reinstate fear/anxiety to the S^D and because fear/anxiety has been reduced effectively in the past by making the avoidance response, the animal's reaction following the punishing/fear-provoking stimulus is to make the same response it had previously learned reduces fear (see Figure 4.2). Importantly, the punishing stimulus need not be in the same modality as

the original aversive stimulus used to establish avoidance responding (e.g., shock can be used to punish an avoidance response established by loud noise and vice versa).[47] Moreover, the tendency for vicious circle behavior to occur is increased when the punishing stimulus is only delivered occasionally (rather than every time the AR is made). Finally, the aversive stimulus need not be delivered contingent on the animal's avoidance response for the vicious circle behavior to occur, that is, noncontingent occurrence of the aversive outcome can also support vicious circle behavior.[48]

Consider the following analogy to what we know about the worry process. Research reviewed above suggests that worry is triggered by some potentially threatening trigger topic or stimulus (or negative automatic thoughts[31]); this occurs in non-anxious as well as anxious people. We will label the trigger topic the S^D (in humans no conditioning of anxiety is generally necessary for this to have threatening meaning, i.e. the first step in Figure 4.1-early is not necessary) and the worry response an avoidance response (AR) based on the research reviewed above by Borkovec et al.[29] This AR is negatively reinforced both because it serves to superstitiously prevent the feared trigger event from occurring and because it helps to escape and/or avoid the sympathetic arousal that might be caused by the trigger topic (for these and other sources of negative reinforcement see Figure 4.3). Thus for most people worry as an avoidance response can be strengthened and the person can potentially gain a sense of perceived control over the trigger situation; in turn, perceived control over aversive situations is also associated with decreased anxiety.[49-51]

But what leads some people to become pathological worriers and receive a diagnosis of GAD? First, as we have seen, worry as an avoidance response (that is somewhat aversive

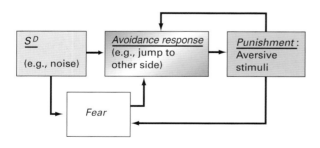

Figure 4.2 Paradoxical effect of punishment on extinction of avoidance learning. Note: Solid line with an arrow indicates one box leads to (or increases the likelihood of) the other.

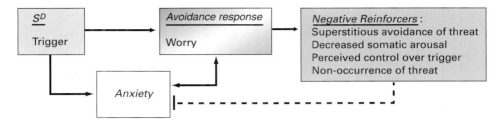

Figure 4.3 The psychological processes that underlie non-pathological worry. Note: Solid line with an arrow indicates one box leads to (or increases the likelihood of) the other. Dashed line with a bar indicates one box inhibits (or decreases the likelihood of) the other.

in nature) sometimes leads to more worry and negative intrusive thoughts which may operate as response-contingent (or not contingent) punishing events (see Figure 4.4). These negative intrusive thoughts may serve as additional trigger topics (S[D]s) which set the occasion for more worry as an AR, both because it has been negatively reinforced in the past by suppression of somatic arousal and superstitious avoidance of the trigger topics and because people expect worry to be useful in these and other ways (see Figure 4.4-upper right). Thus through a positive feedback process the negative intrusive thoughts (punishing stimuli) generated by the initial worry AR come to generate more worry. Because the punishing effects probably do not always occur, the vicious circle that is created is probably especially strong.[46] At the same time the person is likely to develop a sense of perceived inability to control the process of worry (because worry is leading to more worry and more negative intrusive thoughts). (See Figure 4.4-right.) Perceived uncontrollability of worry, in turn, is likely to lead to attempts to control or suppress worry about negative topics. However, as noted earlier, such attempts at control seem to lead to increases in worry and anxiety shortly thereafter. These findings are in keeping with perceived uncon-

trollability of the worry process as being a defining feature of GAD diagnostic criteria. Perceptions of uncontrollability over negative events (such as worry) are also known to generate more anxiety than do comparable negative events that are perceived to be controllable.[50,51] This would provide further input into the vicious circle, especially because, as reviewed earlier, anxiety is known to be associated with an attentional bias toward threat and a negative interpretive bias for ambiguous information. (See Figure 4.4-bottom left.) These additional threatening cues can serve as trigger topics for more anxiety and worry.

In addition, as perceptions of uncontrollability over the worry process develop, and anxiety increases, meta-worry (worry about worry) may begin to develop as a by-product of humans' tendencies to appraise and evaluate topics of personal concern.[35] That is, as the worry process is experienced as being more uncontrollable and intrusive people may begin to worry about the long-term consequences of worry such as having a 'mental breakdown'.[52] In at least several studies meta-worry has been shown to distinguish people with GAD from non-clinical worriers. By contrast, the content of worry about external and non-cognitive internal events often does not distinguish

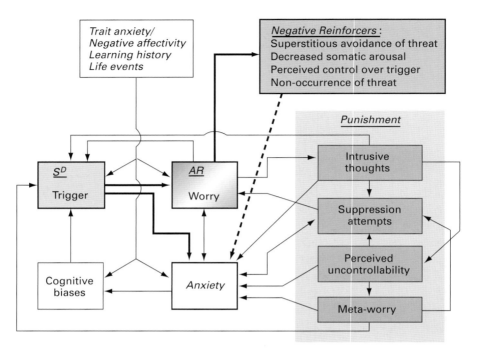

Figure 4.4 The psychological processes that underlie pathological worry in GAD. Note: Bold lines reflect the same processes noted in Figure 4.3 for non-pathological worry. Solid line with an arrow indicates one box leads to (or increases the likelihood of) the other. Dashed line with a bar indicates one box inhibits (or decreases the likelihood of) the other.

people with GAD from normal controls.[31] Wells further argues that as meta-worry develops attempts to try to control the worry increase, but as already noted such attempts often have the paradoxical effect of increasing the frequency of these thoughts (see Figure 4.4-lower right). That meta-worry may make an independent contribution to the pathological worry seen in GAD beyond the perceived uncontrollability of worry is consistent with one questionnaire study showing that meta-worry was associated with pathological worry even when levels of trait anxiety and controllability were accounted for.[52]

Finally we should consider what makes some people more likely than others to get into this vicious circle. As reviewed earlier in

this chapter, people with high trait negative affect (which is likely to be a risk factor for GAD) have an increased tendency to worry, to perceive things as negative (see Figure 4.4-upper left), and to have attentional and interpretive biases. Therefore they are most likely to get into the vicious circle just described. Vicarious learning history (e.g., having a worrier parent) may also contribute to this vicious circle by serving as a distal factor for an increased tendency to worry about things and for perceiving worry as beneficial (see Bouton et al.[53] for a discussion of this kind of risk factor with panic disorder). In addition, distal or proximal factors such as experiencing negative life events provide additional trigger topics (S^{D}s) for the initiation and perpetuation of this circle and may contribute to perceptions of uncontrollability. (See Borkovec et al.[29] for discussion of possible contributions of negative life events to increases in susceptibility to worry and GAD.)

Conclusions

In this chapter we have reviewed a variety of conceptual and etiological issues regarding GAD. We first discussed structural models of anxiety and mood disorders and where GAD lies in this framework. Individuals with GAD are characterized by high levels of negative affectivity, which has led some to conceptualize GAD as an extreme personality trait that places people at risk for other emotional disorders. Others have considered the possibility of conceptualizing GAD as a personality disorder, and this might be indicated for the majority for whom the disorder has an early and chronic course. But for others GAD can start well into adult life and for now GAD remains an Axis I disorder in DSM-IV. Like other Axis I emotional disorders, GAD is characterized by certain cognitive biases, especially attentional biases for threatening information and negative interpretive biases for ambiguous information.[17] These biases provide additional trigger topics for the worry process – the cardinal feature of GAD. Further, we suggested that the normal worry process may be reinforced as a cognitive avoidance response.[29] Then we described how the negative consequences of worry that accrue more or less simultaneously with the positive consequences may lead to a positive feedback process in which worry leads to more worry and anxiety, perceived uncontrollability, and meta-worry. This positive feedback process has been previously described in a somewhat similar manner by others. However, the model we propose goes further by providing a mechanism for how these negative consequences of worry may serve as punishing stimuli that create a vicious circle of more worry. This is analogous to findings in the animal literature that show that punishment of conditioned avoidance responses paradoxically often leads to more avoidance responding rather than less.

References

1. Roemer L, Orsillo SM, Barlow DH Generalized Anxiety Disorder. In Barlow, DH (ed) *Anxiety and its Disorders, Second Edition.* (New York, NY: Guilford Press 2002) 477–515.
2. Kendler KS Major depression and generalised anxiety disorder same genes, (partly) different environments—Revisited, *Br J Psychiatry* (1996) **168**: 68–75.
3. Mineka S, Watson D, Clark LA Comorbidity of anxiety and unipolar mood disorders, *Annu Rev Psychol* (1998) **49**: 377–412.
4. Clark LA, Watson D Tripartite model of anxiety and depression: Psychometric evidence and taxonomic implications, *J Abnorm Psychol* (1991) **100**: 316–36.
5. Brown TA, Chorpita B, Barlow DH Structural relationships among dimensions of the DSM-IV anxiety and mood disorders and dimensions of negative affect, positive affect, and autonomic arousal, *J Abnorm Psychol* (1998) **107**: 179–92.
6. Watson D, Clark LA, Weber K, Assenheimer JS Testing a tripartite model: II. Exploring the symptom structure of anxiety and depression in student, adult, and patient samples, *J Abnorm Psychol* (1995) **104**: 15–25.
7. Borkovec TD, Lyonfields JD, Wiser SL, Deihl L The role of worrisome thinking in the suppression of cardiovascular response to phobic imagery, *Behav Res Ther* (1993) **31**: 321–4.

8. Brown TA, Di Nardo PA, Lehman CL, Campbell LA, Reliability of DSM-IV anxiety and mood disorders: Implications for the classification of emotional disorders, *J Abnorm Psychol* (2001) **110**: 49–58.

9. Krueger RF, Caspi A, Moffitt TE, Silva P et al., Personality traits are differentially linked to mental disorders: A multitrait-multidiagnosis study of an adolescent birth cohort, *J Abnorm Psychol* (1996) **105**: 299–312.

10. Clark LA, Watson D, Mineka S, Temperament, personality, and the mood and anxiety disorders, *J Abnorm Psychol* (1994) **103**: 103–16.

11. Brown TA, The nature of generalized anxiety disorder and pathological worry: Current evidence and conceptual models, *Can J Psychiatry* (1997) **42**: 817–25.

12. Sanderson WC, Barlow DH, A description of patients diagnosed with DSM-III-R generalized anxiety disorder, *J Nerv Ment Dis* (1990) **178**: 588–91

13. Blazer D, Hughes D, George LK, Stressful life events and the onset of a generalized anxiety syndrome, *Am J Psychiatry,* (1987) **144**:1178–83.

14. Craske MG, Rapee RM, Jackel L, Barlow DH, Qualitative dimensions of worry in DSM-III-R generalized anxiety disorder subjects and nonanxious controls, *Behav Res Ther* (1989) **27**: 397–402.

15. Barlow DH, Di Nardo PA, The diagnosis of generalized anxiety disorder: Development, current status, and future directions. In Rapee RM, Barlow DH, (eds), *Chronic anxiety: Generalized anxiety disorder and mixed anxiety-depression.* (New York, NY The Guilford Press: 1991) 95–118.

16. Mineka S, Tomarken AJ, The role of cognitive biases in the origins and maintenance of fear and anxiety disorders. In Archer T, Nilsson L-G (eds) *Aversion, avoidance, and anxiety: Perspectives on aversively motivated behavior* (Hillsdale, NJ: Lawrence Erlbaum 1989) 195–221.

17. Mineka S, Rafaeli E, Yovel I, Cognitive biases in emotional disorders: Social-cognitive and information processing perspectives. In Davidson R, Goldsmith H, Scherer K, (eds) *Handbook of Affective Science* (Oxford University Press 2002).

18. Williams JM, Watts FN, MacLeod C, Mathews A, *Cognitive psychology and emotional disorders,* 2nd edn (Chichester: Wiley 1997).

19. Mathews A, MacLeod C Cognitive approaches to emotion and emotional disorders, *Annu Rev Psychol* (1994) **45**: 25–50.

20. MacLeod C Anxiety and anxiety disorders. In: Dalgleish T, Power, MJ, eds, *Handbook of cognition and emotion* (Chichester: Wiley 1999) 447–77.

21. Mathews A, Mogg K, Kentish J, Eysenck M Effect of psychological treatment on cognitive bias in generalized anxiety disorder, *Behav Res Ther* (1995) **33**: 293–303.

22. Mogg K, Bradley BP, Millar N, White J A follow-up study of cognitive bias in generalized anxiety disorder, *Behav Res Ther* (1995) **33**: 927–35.

23. MacLeod C, Hagan R Individual differences in the selective processing of threatening information, and emotional responses to a stressful life event, *Behav Res Ther* (1992) **30**: 151–61.

24. Pury CLS, Information processing predictors of emotional response to stress, *Cognition and Emotion* (in press)

25. MacLeod AK Prospective cognitions. In: Dalgleish T, Power MJ, eds, *Handbook of Cognition and Emotion* (Chichester: Wiley 1999) 267–80.

26. Eysenck MW, Mogg K, May J, Richards A, Mathews A Bias in interpretation of ambiguous sentences related to threat in anxiety, *J Abnorm Psychol* (1991) **100**: 144–50.

27. Mathews A, Mackintosh B Induced emotional interpretation bias and anxiety, *J Abnorm Psychol* (2000) **109**: 602–15.

28. Borkovec TD The nature, functions, and origins of worry. In Davey GCL, Tallis F, (eds) *Worrying: Perspectives on theory, assessment and treatment* (New York: Wiley 1994) 5–33.

29. Borkovec TD, Alcaine O, Behar E Avoidance theory of worry and generalized anxiety disorder. In Heimberg RG, Turk CL, Mennin DS (eds) *Generalized anxiety disorder: Advances in research and practice* (New York: Guilford Press in press).

30. Wells A, Meta-cognition and worry: A cognitive model of generalized anxiety disorder, *Behavioural & Cognitive Psychotherapy* (1995) **23**: 301–320.

31. Wells A A cognitive model of generalized anxiety disorder, *Behav Modif* (1999) **23**: 526–55.

32. Dugas MJ, Gagnon F, Ladouceur R, Freeston MH, Generalized anxiety disorder: A preliminary test of a conceptual model, *Behav Res Ther* (1998) **36**: 215–26.

33. Foa EB, Kozak MJ, Emotional processing of fear: Exposure to corrective information, *Psychol Bull* (1986) **99**: 20–35.

34. Borkovec TD, Hazlett-Stevens H, Diaz ML, The role of positive beliefs about worry in generalized anxiety disorder and its treatment, *Clin Psychol Psychotherapy* (1999) **6**:126–38.

35. Wells A, Butler G, Generalized anxiety disorder. In Clark DM, Fairburn CG (eds) *Science and practice of cognitive behaviour therapy* (New York: Oxford University Press 1997) 155–78.

36. Wells A, Papageorgiou C, Worry and the incubation of intrusive images following stress, *Behav Res Ther* (1995) 33: 579–83.

37. Butler G, Wells A, Dewick H, Differential effects of worry and imagery after exposure to a stressful stimulus: A pilot study, *Behavioural & Cognitive Psychotherapy* (1995) 23: 45–56.

38. Roemer L, Borkovec TD, Effects of suppressing thoughts about emotional material, *J Abnormal Psychol* (1994) 103: 467–74.

39. Purdon C, Thought suppression and psychopathology, *Behav Res Ther* (1999) 37: 129–54.

40. Wenzlaff RM, Wegner DM, Roper DW, Depression and mental control: The resurgence of unwanted negative thoughts, *J Pers Soc Psychol* (1988) 55: 882–92.

41. Salkovskis PM, Campbell P, Thought suppression induces intrusion in naturally occurring negative intrusive thoughts, *Behav Res Ther* (1994) 32: 1–8.

42. Dean SJ, Pittman CM, Self-punitive behavior: A revised analysis. In Denny MR, ed, *Fear, avoidance, and phobias: A fundamental analysis* (Hillsdale, NJ: Lawrence Erlbaum Associates 1991) 259–84.

43. Mineka S, The role of fear in theories of avoidance learning, flooding, and extinction, *Psychol Bull* (1979) 86: 985–1010.

44. Solomon RL, Kamin LJ, Wynne LC, Traumatic avoidance learning: The outcomes of several extinction procedures with dogs, *J Abnorm Psychol* (1953) 48: 291–302.

45. Seligman MEP, Johnston J, A cognitive theory of avoidance learning. In McGuigan FS, Lumsden D (eds) *Contemporary approaches to conditioning and learning* (Washington, DC: V.H. Winston & Sons 1973).

46. Brown JS, Factors affecting self-punitive locomotor behavior. In Campbell B, Church R (eds) *Punishment and Aversive Behavior* (New York: Appleton Century Crofts 1969) 467–514.

47. Melvin KB, Martin RC, Facilitative effects of two modes of punishment on resistance to extinction, *Journal of Comparative & Physiological Psychology* (1966) 62: 491–4.

48. Mackintosh NJ, *The psychology of animal learning* (New York: Academic Press 1974)

49. Cook M, Mineka S, Trumble D, The role of response-produced and exteroceptive feedback in the attenuation of fear over the course of avoidance learning, *J Exp Psychol Anim Behav Process* (1987) 13: 239–49.

50. Mineka S, Zinbarg R, Conditioning and ethological models of anxiety disorders: Stress-in-Dynamic-Context Anxiety models. In Hope DA (ed) *Nebraska Symposium on Motivation, 1995: Perspectives on anxiety, panic, and fear. Current theory and research in motivation, 43* (Lincoln, NE: University of Nebraska Press 1996) 135–210.

51. Sanderson WC, Rapee RM, Barlow DH, The influence of an illusion of control on panic attacks induced via inhalation of 5.5% carbon dioxide-enriched air, *Arch Gen Psychiatry* (1989) 46: 157–62.

52. Wells A, Carter K, Preliminary tests of a cognitive model of generalized anxiety disorder, *Behav Res Ther* (1999) 37: 585–94.

53. Bouton ME, Mineka S, Barlow DH, A modern learning theory perspective on the etiology of panic disorder, *Psychol Rev* (2001) 108: 4–32.

II   Pathogenesis

5

The Neurobiology of Generalized Anxiety Disorder

David J Nutt and Jayne E Bailey

The brain mechanisms or neurobiology of generalized anxiety disorder (GAD) can be considered under two main headings – the neurotransmitter mechanisms that underpin the symptoms and signs of the syndrome and the brain circuits that mediate these.

The brain circuits of GAD

Brain circuitry can be explored in a number of ways but in recent years the main approach has been the use of neuroimaging techniques, especially PET and SPECT and now fMRI. The few studies so far have been limited to PET, and both oxygen 15 and 18F-deoxyglucose measures have been made.[1,2] Although the results are limited and somewhat contradictory, they have suggested that underlying GAD is a neuronal circuit that incorporates several areas of cortex plus the basal ganglia and parts of the limbic system and thalamus. These can be integrated into a circuit diagram as in Figure 5.1 which attempts to relate the brain regions implicated in GAD with the

symptoms and signs of the disorder (see also Nutt[3]). The potential role of neurotransmitters in each region is discussed below.

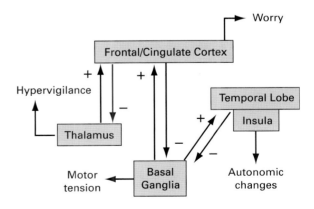

Figure 5.1: Schematic representation of brain regions that might generate symptoms and signs of GAD. + and − represent the usual direction of stimulatory and inhibitory control respectively. In GAD the drive from basal ganglia to cortex may be overactive and/or the descending inhibitory control underactive, so leading to an overactive cortex/basal ganglia loop as is also seen in OCD

Of some interest is the relation between these observations and those found in depression and other anxiety disorders. There is some overlap in the regions involved in depression and GAD (reviewed in Nutt[3]) but the direction of effect may vary. Obsessive-compulsive disorder (OCD) and GAD may share features in that there is evidence for an overactive fronto-cortical–basal ganglial loop in both conditions, and it is possible that antidepressants serve to decrease this overactivity in both conditions. However, many studies in OCD have shown that the overactive loop is one from the orbitofrontal cortex to the basal ganglia[4] whereas in GAD it is from more rostral parts of the frontal cortex, which accounts for some of the main symptom differences between the two disorders. Evidence for thalamic involvement accords with the recent data that this brain region is involved in attention, probably through a noradrenergic input.[5]

Neurotransmitter function and GAD

Brain neurotransmitter function is rather more difficult to study directly, especially in psychiatric disorders where brain biopsies are not feasible and very few subjects commit suicide so post mortem studies are not available. In essence, this situation is one that pertains to all the anxiety disorders, and the alternative strategies that can be used to address this question are listed in Table 5.1. They include very proxy measures such as plasma and urine assays as well as more direct interventions that involve the administration of drugs or other challenges that target known brain mechanisms and whose output can be measured easily.

Table 5.1: Approaches to the neurochemistry of GAD

- Peripheral measures
    e.g. plasma / urine NA, A, MHPG
- CSF measures
    e.g. NA, MHPG, 5HIAA, opioid peptides, DBI
- Receptor sensitivity - challenge tests
    e.g. clonidine / yohimbine – α_2 receptors
    mCPP / L-tryptophan – 5HT receptors
    benzodiazepines – benzo receptors
    CRF – CRF receptors
- Post mortem studies
    transmitters and receptors
- Cerebral blood flow
    PET, SPECT, fMRI
- Receptor studies – PET and SPECT
    $GABA_A$ receptors
    $5HT_{1A}$, $5HT_2$ receptors and uptake sites
    dopamine receptors and uptake sites
    NA peripheral transporter

Although there are a number of these different approaches that have been used in the anxiety disorders, studies in GAD are extremely limited. This reflects the fact that GAD has for so long been a Cinderella syndrome and one that does not greatly impinge on the research psychiatrist who has been involved in studies of the other major anxiety disorders. Also in other psychiatric disorders post mortem studies have proved instructive but as GAD patients rarely commit suicide there appear to have been none conducted for this disorder.

Interest in the biology of GAD is in the process of changing consequent on the growing interest in the use of the SSRIs and venlafaxine in the treatment of this disorder. We can presume that there will be a significant growth in biological research in GAD over the next ten years.

Table 5.2: Theories of GAD derived from treatment studies

Treatment	Theory	Evidence?
Benzodiazepines	Decreased GABA-A receptor function Endogenous inverse agonist	Decreased binding in SPECT study Not yet
Buspirone	? Increased presynaptic 5HT activity ? Decreased postsynaptic 5HT function	? ?
SSRIs	Decreased postsynaptic 5HT function Receptor sensitivity change	? Possible
Hydroxyzine	Increased histamine H1 receptor stimulation	Not yet
SNRIs	Decreased NA function	Yes – decreased clonidine responses
Trazodone	? Altered NA or 5HT function	Yes – decreased clonidine responses

Another approach to the question of neurobiology relates to the issue of how treatments of GAD or other psychiatric disorders work. Back extrapolation from a knowledge of treatment effects has proved a fruitful way of at least generating testable hypotheses about a number of psychiatric disorders. Perhaps the most obvious is the dopamine theory of schizophrenia which emerged from an insight into the strong correlation between the affinity of the effective treatments, the neuroleptics and the doses used in clinical treatment. From this classic correlation plot came the idea that schizophrenia was a disorder of dopamine receptors which has, in a modified form, stood the test of time although there have been many doubters.[6] If we apply the same strategy to GAD we can immediately generate a number of hypotheses, as in Table 5.2, because there are a number of different drug treatments for this disorder.

What can we learn from the challenge and other studies that have been conducted so far?

GABA *receptor function*

This is a straightforward functional theory that can relate to GAD as well as, if not better than, any of the anxiety disorders. In its simplest form it states that there is a relative deficiency of GABA-A function in the brains of patients with GAD that leads to anxiety. The evidence for this comes from the proven effect of the benzodiazepines in GAD and the growing knowledge of the mechanism of action of these drugs. The benzodiazepines we know act as direct and immediate modulators of brain GABA function and there is a vast body of data linking GABA to anxiety both in animals and humans.[7] A plot of GABA-A receptor affinity against clinical dose (Figure 5.2) shows that there is an excellent correlation between the two, which further supports the evaluation of this receptor system as a potential aetiological or pathological mechanism.

There are essentially two theories that translate from this observation: the first says

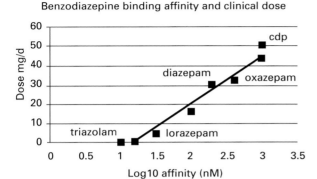

Figure 5.2: Correlation of benzodiazepine binding affinity and clinical dose. cdp = chlordiazepoxide

that the GABA-A receptor is down-regulated or sub-functioning; and the other postulates that there is an endogenous anxiogenic substance that acts to decrease GABA-A receptor function in the manner of an inverse agonist. There is already one study that supports a receptor-based theory – Tiihonen and colleagues[8] in Finland using a new iodine 123-labelled SPECT tracer 123-I-NNM to study a group of GAD patients found decreased binding in the left temporal pole. There are other radiotracers for the GABA-A receptor, especially the PET tracer 11C-flumazenil and the SPECT tracer 123-I iomazenil. As yet there are no studies reported with these tracers in GAD, although our own group has found that there is a significant reduction in flumazenil binding in panic disorder patients.[9] These patients showed a much more widely distributed down-regulation of GABA-A receptor binding compared with the limited reduction seen in the patients in the GAD study. This is consistent with the general position that the panic disorder patients are more anxious and have a more acutely severe form of anxiety than those with GAD.

The alternative theory is that in GAD patients there exists in the brain a naturally occurring or endogenous inverse agonist of the benzodiazepine receptor. Inverse agonists are substances that act in exactly the opposite manner to benzodiazepine agonists in that they are anxiogenic as well as proconvulsant and sleep-reducing.[10] There have been many of these substances synthesized, and there are some suggestions from animal studies that endogenous ones might be present based on the fact that the benzodiazepine antagonist flumazenil can have anxiolytic properties.[11] This sort of approach would be perhaps the best method of resolving whether such a substance mediates GAD, since if one was active then its effects would be blocked by flumazenil. We took an equivalent approach in the case of panic disorder and to our surprise found that flumazenil was anxiogenic rather than anxiolytic.[10,12] Strangely, despite flumazenil being available as a research tool for over a decade, this sort of approach has not yet been used in GAD, although it has in other anxiety disorders such as post-traumatic stress disorder[11] and premenstrual dysphoric disorder.[13] Again, this may reflect the low priority given to GAD in the minds of researchers or funding bodies. If flumazenil was anxiolytic this would not only be of some scientific interest but could also lead to a new treatment strategy. Antagonists have real advantages over agonists in that they do not produce dependence or withdrawal and have much reduced sedative or other side effects.

One final point needs to be made about the benzodiazepine receptor in anxiety. There is now extensive evidence about the nature and distribution of GABA-A receptor subtypes and the actions of GABA in the brain that they mediate.[10] It now seems that the α_2 and the α_3 subtypes of the receptor are the most likely to be implicated in anxiety, whereas the α_1 subtype tends to mediate sedation. New drugs targeting these receptor subtypes are in development and we may soon know if they do work in animal models of GAD. The α_5 subtype is found in high density in the hippocampus and is known to be involved in memory. However, we have recently developed a PET tracer for this subtype and have found that in humans it is also located in other limbic regions, especially the anterior cingulate cortex, the ventral striatum and other parts of the temporal lobe including the amygdala.[14] It would be interesting to know if the Tiihonen et al findings could reflect a change in specific subunits,[8] although it is not known what the receptor subtype pharmacology of the 123-I-NNM SPECT tracer is.

5HT

The role of 5HT in anxiety is a complex one.[15] There are data that suggest that an increase in 5HT mediates anxiety and there is contradictory evidence that 5HT is anxiolytic (see also Chapter 8). Similarly for 5HT-acting drugs such as the SSRIs and buspirone it is not known whether they act to increase 5HT function directly or indirectly, or rather produce some sort of receptor adaptation or down-regulation.

One way of resolving these issues is to consider that there might be two forms of anxiety. One, conditioned anxiety, is targeted to external cues, such as is seen in panic with agoraphobic avoidance of situations in which the anxiety occurs. The other form of anxiety is unconditioned anxiety, such as is seen in innate fears. Deakin and Graeff have detailed the theory behind this and speculated that 5HT might help restrain unconditioned anxiety whereas it might worsen the conditioned

form.[16] Testing this theory is not simple. One approach is to use challenge tests with 5HT agonists such as mCPP. This has been done in a group of GAD patients who reported an increase in subjective anxiety that was significantly greater than that seen in the control group, suggesting more reactive 5HT receptors.[17] Interpreting these findings is complicated, however, given the marked baseline differences between the groups, the GAD patients being much more anxious at baseline than the control group. Indeed, if the subjective anxiety following the mCPP is presented as a percentage change score from this baseline then the volunteers have a much higher response than the patients. Such issues of interpretation bedevil such challenge studies.

An alternative strategy is to consider whether there are measurable differences in 5HT receptor number using imaging techniques. Tracers for 5HT receptor subtypes are now available and one, 11C-WAY 100635, which labels the 5HT 1A receptor, has been used in both depression and in panic disorder. In both these disorders it has been found that there is a generalized decrease in 5HT receptor binding.[18,19] It would therefore be timely to extend these studies to GAD quite soon. Moreover, in view of the proven efficacy of buspirone in GAD, a knowledge of the baseline 5HT 1A receptor measures might help resolve the complicated question of how this drug actually works.

Another somewhat more direct approach to 5HT function in anxiety is to manipulate 5HT function quite directly. This can be done using the technique of tryptophan depletion, which reduces 5HT synaptic function by decreasing the availability of the precursor amino acid l-tryptophan. This technique has been used increasingly in recent years and has enabled major insights into the biology of many psychiatric disorders.[20] There have been no studies in GAD as yet, but in other anxiety disorders there is evidence that reducing 5HT is somewhat anxiogenic.[21]

This technique can also give important insights into the actions of treatments. For example, in depression it has been clearly demonstrated that tryptophan depletion will undermine or abolish the antidepressant action of drugs that act on the 5HT system such as the SSRIs and the MAOIs, whereas it was without effect in patients who had been effectively treated with an antidepressant that acted on the noradrenaline system.[22] Conversely a manipulation that reduced noradrenaline function (the synthesis inhibitor αMPT) undid the antidepressant action of noradrenaline-acting drugs such as desipramine but had no effect on the antidepressant action of 5HT-acting drugs. There is less work in the anxiety disorders, but our own group has shown that the anti-panic action of the SSRIs can be undone by tryptophan depletion.[23,24] In this study a challenge with flumazenil was used to induce panic during the period of maximal 5HT depletion and it is likely that this was critical to the observed finding since before the panic challenge the changes in anxiety were less pronounced. In OCD a tryptophan depletion study did not reveal much difference,[25] which could suggest that the mode of action of the SSRIs is rather different between these two disorders.

However, it may be that one needs to provoke anxiety in the experimental situation in order to maximize the observed tryptophan depletion action. This is relevant to the investigation of GAD, where it would be easy to conduct such a study but a false negative might emerge. Perhaps we should be working towards developing a simple psychological challenge to provoke GAD symptoms in patients undergoing such procedures.

Noradrenaline

The nature and distribution of the central noradrenaline system, especially that originating from the locus coeruleus, makes this a reasonable candidate for involvement in GAD. Noradrenaline neuronal firing is very stress-sensitive and can be conditioned to fearful stimuli. Moreover, noradrenaline is involved in attentional processing and there is evidence for attentional bias in GAD (Chapter 4). Plasma noradrenaline concentrations offer a proxy measure of brain noradrenaline activity, and these have been shown to be somewhat elevated in GAD but not to the same extent as in depression.[26] As yet there are no good measures of central noradrenaline and no imaging probes have been developed. We must therefore rely on studies using challenges with noradrenaline agonists such as clonidine (see below). In principle, challenges with α_2-adrenoceptor antagonists such as idazoxan,[27] would also be useful but none have been reported in GAD patients.

Clonidine is an α_2-adrenoceptor agonist that can be used to assess the sensitivity of the central α_2-adrenoceptor. The dependent measures that clonidine will influence range from endocrine release, especially growth hormone and hypothermia, through to hypotension and REM sleep suppression. In GAD there have been only a couple of studies reported. One from the group in Ann Arbor examined the endocrine effects of clonidine and found that GAD patients showed reduced release compared with normal volunteers, in fact they had a similar response to the group of depressed patients also studied.[28] In this regard GAD patients resemble those with panic disorder, who also have reduced growth hormone responses to clonidine.[29] One explanation for this general finding is that all three conditions are associated with increased central noradrenaline release secondary to stress. This elevated noradrenaline release would then lead to a down-regulation of post-synaptic α_2-adreno-ceptors. If this were the case, then we would presume that successful treatment would rectify the blunted hormonal response, but studies on this have not yet been conducted. It would be important to perform such a study using either a benzodiazepine or psychological therapy, as both antidepressants and buspirone can affect α_2-adrenoceptor function.

The other measure of α_2-adrenoceptor sensitivity in GAD is the REM sleep suppression test. This relies on the fact that REM sleep is very sensitive to clonidine, which will delay its expression in a dose-related way. In depression the effects of clonidine are quite blunted, and Schittecatte and colleagues[30] conducted a direct comparison of GAD and depressed patients using sleep lab monitoring and clonidine administration after the first REM sleep period. They confirmed their own previous finding that clonidine markedly suppressed REM in normal volunteers – in this study it doubled the period from the first to second REM sleep periods. In the depressed group this effect was almost absent, whereas the GAD patients had a profile indistinguishable from the volunteers.[30]

Taken together, these findings with clonidine do not support a view that there is a general dysfunction of central α_2-adrenoceptors in GAD although it is possible that localized abnormalities exist. Our own studies are currently using the clonidine challenge paradigm in GAD to examine its effects on central executive function and regional cerebral blood flow as shown on SPECT.

Histamine

The efficacy of hydroxyzine and, to a lesser extent, other antihistamines in GAD (Chapter 3) might lead one to suspect that this transmitter could be involved in GAD. Our knowledge of the role of histamine in the brain is still rather rudimentary but it does seem to promote wakefulness and may increase attention. The main target of the antihistamine drugs for GAD are the histamine H1 receptors which are found throughout the brain and mediate the sedative side effects of many drugs, including the older neuroleptics such as chlorpromazine and the tricyclic antidepressants. There is no evidence yet that brain histamine is overactive in GAD, or indeed in any disorder, so we presume that the action of the antihistamines is to produce a degree of central sedation that may in itself be anxiolytic but might also interfere with the attentional biases found in GAD.

Dopamine

Finally we should briefly mention dopamine as there is quite a tradition of using neuroleptics to treat anxiety even though the majority of these drugs do not have either a licence or any good clinical trial evidence for this indication.[31] In fact in the UK the only neuroleptic licensed for this sort of indication is low dose flupenthixol ("Fluanxol") although in many other European countries low dose sulpiride is also licensed for anxiety. These drugs are thought to act predominantly by blocking the dopamine D2 receptor, which suggests that dopamine systems might play a role in GAD. The PET finding that the basal ganglia may show altered activity in GAD[1] supports this idea, and we have suggested that basal ganglia overactivity might contribute to the motor symptoms of GAD (see Figure 5.1). It would be of interest to explore whether these symptoms were preferentially affected by drugs such as flupenthixol. Also of note are the observations of dopamine D2 receptor

PET[32] and dopamine transporter SPECT[33] abnormalities in another major anxiety disorder – social anxiety disorder. These sorts of neuroimaging studies would bear repeating in GAD.

Integrating neurochemistry and brain circuits of GAD

A biological theory of GAD should ideally incorporate facts relating to brain chemistry with those defining brain circuits. We have attempted to do this in Figure 5.3. This shows the brain regions that seem at present to be involved in GAD with the possible neurotransmitters that might contribute to the abnormality. Upon this we have then suggested where might be the main sites of action of the various different drug classes that are effective in GAD.

It is likely that within the next decade it will be possible to directly test these ideas

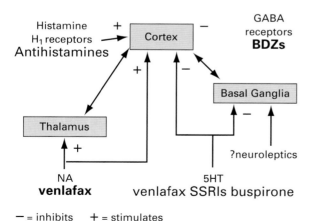

− = inhibits   + = stimulates

Figure 5.3: Possible sites of action of effective treatments of GAD

using targeted PET or SPECT probes for the specific receptors in the particular brain regions. Moreover, the development of the new technique of pharmaco-fMRI, which should allow the site of drug effects to be visualized, may make it possible to directly estimate the brain sites at which drugs act to modify specific symptoms and signs of GAD.

Is it possible to model GAD in human volunteers?

Human volunteer models can make a useful contribution to understanding the brain mechanisms of a number of psychiatric disorders and may also allow the rapid screening of new potential therapeutic agents. In the anxiety field there have been many approaches to anxiety induction, which range from naturalistic fears such as experienced during parachute jumps through to public speaking and the threat of painful shocks. It is not clear which if any of these might be a valid model for GAD. Our own study of anticipatory anxiety in a fear-conditioned paradigm found that the anxiety induced by anticipation of an electric shock was both reliably induced and amenable to attenuation by the benzodiazepine midazolam given intravenously.[10] We also found using 15-O water PET that the anxiety was linked with changes in blood flow in a number of parts of the limbic circuit and frontal cortical regions.[34] However, it is uncertain whether such conditioned fear models do model GAD despite their apparent sensitivity to benzodiazepines. For this reason we have explored the use of carbon dioxide (CO_2) as an anxiogenic provocation.

CO_2 has been used for several decades as a means of provoking unconditioned anxiety.[35] It is a profound stimulus to brainstem

Table 5.3: Comparison of change from baseline values in subjective mood state in response to inhalation of CO_2, as measured by visual analogue scales (0=not at all, 100=the most ever)

Mood state	Our data 7.5% CO_2, n= 8 mean (± sem)	Woods et al[38] 7.5% CO_2, n=8 mean (± sem)	Woods et al[38] 5% CO_2, n=11 (mean (± sem)
Anxious	33 (9)	41 (8)	14 (7)
Fearful	31 (8)	30 (9)	3 (2)
Relaxed/Calm*	−46 (3)	−31 (7)	−9 (6)
Happy	−35 (5)	−13 (5)	−2 (6)
* our study used 'relaxed', Woods used 'calm'.			

chemoreceptors which are thought to activate a wide range of higher brain structures that lead to physiological activation plus escape behaviour. In recent years CO_2 models have generally involved the breathing of a single or double vital capacity inhalation of 35% CO_2 mixture, or 5% CO_2 for 15–20 minute duration. Both procedures cause acute severe anxiety in patients with panic disorder, which is very similar to spontaneously occurring panic attacks,[36] but in healthy volunteers both concentrations of CO_2 produce subjective anxiety to a lesser degree. However, we have recently found that a vital capacity inhalation of 35% CO_2 will increase subjective fear and produce a measurable activation of the hypothalamo-pituitary adrenal axis stress response by increasing plasma cortisol levels in normal volunteers.[37]

Using a concentration of 7.5% CO_2 delivered over a longer time gives a different picture, which is one of a rise in anxiety associated with increased autonomic arousal, feelings of tension and a reduction in the sense of being relaxed. These responses thus generated last for the duration of the period of inhalation, which can be as long as 20 minutes[38,39] and subjects report significantly greater anxiety than with the 5% CO_2 inhalation (Table 5.3).

We have been developing a paradigm of anxiety which is based on the continual breathing of 7.5% CO_2 in air, and an example of the time course of the changes in feeling relaxed (measured by visual analogue rating scales) produced by this as compared with a single breath of 35% CO_2 is shown in Figure 5.4. Moreover, an analysis of the symptoms produced by the two contrasting paradigms shows that the 35% CO_2 produces a profile that mimics a panic attack whereas 7.5% CO_2 produces symptoms that are more GAD-like (Table 5.4).

Of course the critical issue is now whether this CO_2 model is a valid proxy for GAD. Probably the best way of testing this is to prove that treatments that are efficacious in GAD also work in the model. To this end we have studied the actions of the benzodiazepine lorazepam (1mg po) on the subjective and objective symptoms produced by inhalation of 7.5% CO_2 in healthy non-anxious volunteers.

Table 5.4: Percent of subjects reporting panic symptom inventory (PSI) items in response to CO_2 inhalation. Highlighted sections represent differences in response to 7.5% CO_2 with and without lorazepam

PSI Item	35% CO_2 (n=14)	7.5% CO_2 (n=8)	LZP + 7.5% CO_2 (n=9)
Breathlessness	93	88	89
Weakness	79	88	56
Anxiety	71	88	78
Apprehension/Fear	71	88	33
Dizziness	57	88	56
Heart racing	64	75	67
Shakiness	36	75	22
Sweating	29	75	33
Tension	29	75	56
Feelings of unreality	50	63	67
Discomfort in chest	29	63	33
Tight muscles	14	50	33
Fear of loss of control	50	25	44
Fear of going mad	14	25	11
Fear of dying	7	13	0

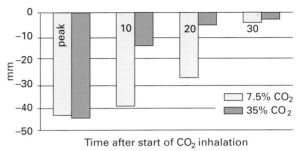

Change from baseline - VAS relaxed

Figure 5.4: Change from baseline in feelings of "relaxed" as measured by visual analogue scale (0=not at all, 100=most ever). N=8 7.5%, N=14 35%

the panic symptom inventory, specifically apprehension and fear, tremor, shakiness, muscle pain and tension – symptoms commonly associated with GAD (Table 5.4).

To further explore whether the inhalation of 7.5% CO_2 will be a model of GAD, it is important to conduct further studies which must include an investigation of the effects of other treatments with proven treatment value in GAD, such as antidepressants (SSRIs and venlafaxine) and buspirone. If we are able to validate this human model then it can be used to explore the neurobiology of GAD and may offer a quick way of exploring the potential therapeutic value of new agents for the treatment of anxiety.

A preliminary analysis of this data suggests that lorazepam reduces some of the symptoms produced by the inhalation, as measured on

References

1. Buchsbaum MS, Wu J, Haier R, et al, Positron emission tomography assessment of effects of benzodiazepines on regional glucose metabolic rate in patients with anxiety disorder, *Life Sci* (1987) 40:2393–400.
2. Wu JC, Buchsbaum MS, Hershey TG, et al, PET in generalized anxiety disorder. *Biol Psychiatry* (1991) 29:1181–9
3. Nutt DJ, Neurobiological mechanisms in generalized anxiety disorder, *J Clin Psychiatry* (2000) 162 (Suppl 11):22–7.
4. Malizia AL, What do brain imaging studies tell us about anxiety disorders? *J Psychopharmacol* (1999) 13:372–8.
5. Coull JT, Buchel C, Friston KJ, et al, Noradrenergically mediated plasticity in a human attentional neuronal network, *Neuroimage* (1999) 10:705–15

6. Laruelle M, Abi-Dargham A, Dopamine as the wind of the psychotic fire: new evidence from brain imaging studies, *J Psychopharmacol* (1999) **13**: 358-71

7. Kalueff A, Nutt DJ, Role of GABA in memory and anxiety, *Depress Anxiety* (1997) **4**:100–10.

8. Tiihonen J, Kuikka J, Rasanen P, et al, Cerebral benzodiazepine receptor binding and distribution in generalized anxiety disorder: a fractional analysis, *Mol Psychiatry* (1997) **2**:463–71.

9. Malizia AL, Cunningham VJ, Bell CM et al, Decreased brain GABAA-benzodiazepine receptor binding in panic disorder preliminary results form a quantitative PET study, *Arch Gen Psychiatry* (1998) **55**:715–20.

10. Nutt DJ, Malizia AL, New insights into the role of the GABA-A-benzodiazepine receptor in psychiatric disorder, *B J Psychiatry* (2001) **179**:390–6.

11. Coupland NJ, Lillywhite A, Bell CJ, Potokar JP, Nutt DJ, A pilot controlled study of the effects of flumazenil in post traumatic stress disorder, *Biol Psychiatry* (1997) **41**:988–90.

12. Nutt DJ, Glue P, Lawson CW, Wilson SJ, Flumazenil provocation of panic attacks: Evidence for altered benzodiazepine receptor sensitivity in panic disorder, *Arch Gen Psychiatry* (1990) **47**: 917–25.

13. Le Melledo JM, Van Driel M, Coupland NJ, Lott P, Jhangri GS, Response to flumazenil in women with premenstrual dysphoric disorder, *Am J Psychiatry* (2000) **157**:821–3

14. Lingford-Hughes A, Hume SP, Feeney A, Hirani E, Osman S, Cunningham VJ, Pike VW, Brooks DJ, Nutt DJ, Imaging the α5-subunit containing GABA-benzodiazepine receptor subtype *In Vivo* with PET, *J Psychopharmacol* (2001) Suppl to 15:A64, K4.

15. Bell CJ, Nutt DJ, Serotonin and panic, *B J Psychiatry* (1998) **172**: 465–471.

16. Deakin JFW, Graeff FG, 5-HT and mechanisms of defence, *J Psychopharmacol* (1991) **5**:305–15.

17. Germine M, Goddard AW, Woods SW, et al, Anger and anxiety responses to m-chlorophenylpiperazine in generalized anxiety disorder, *Biol Psychiatry* (1992) **32**:457–61.

18. Sargent PA, Kjaer KH, Bench CJ, Rabiner EA, Messa C, Meyer J, Gunn RN, Grasby PM, Cowen PJ, Brain serotonin1A receptor binding measured by positron emission tomography with [11C]WAY-100635: effects of depression and antidepressant treatment, *Arch Gen Psychiatry* (2000) **57**:174–80.

19. Sargent PA, Nash J, Hood S, Rabiner E, Messa C, Cowen P, Nutt DJ, Grasby PM, 5-HT1A receptor binding in panic disorder; comparison with depressive disorder and healthy volunteers using PET and [11C]WAY-100635, *Neuroimage* (2000) **11**:189.

20. Bell C, Abrams J, Nutt DJ, Tryptophan depletion and its implications for psychiatry, *Br J Psychiatry* (2001) **178**: 399–405

21. Miller HEJ, Deakin JFW, Anderson I, Effect of acute tryptophan depletion on CO_2 induced anxiety in patients with panic disorder and normal volunteers, *Br J Psychiatry* (2000) **176**: 182–8.

22. Delgado P, Price LH, Miller HL, et al, Serotonin and the neurobiology of depression. *Arch Gen Psychiatry* (1994) **51**:865–74.

23. Nutt DJ, Forshall S, Bell C, et al, Mechanisms of action of selective serotonin reuptake inhibitors in the treatment of psychiatric disorders, *Eur Neuropsychopharmacol* (1999) **9**:S81–S86

24. Bell C, Forshall S, Adrover M, Nash J, Hood S, Argyropoulos S, Rich A, Nutt DJ, Does 5-HT restrain panic? A tryptophan depletion study in panic disorder patients recovered on paroxetine, *J Psychopharmacol* (2002) **16**:5–14.

25. Barr LC, Goodman WK, McDougle CJ, et al, Tryptophan depletion in patients with obsessive-compulsive disorder who respond to serotonin reuptake inhibitors, *Arch Gen Psychiatry* (1994) **51**: 309–17.

26. Kelly CB, Cooper SJ, Differences in variability in plasma noradrenaline between depressive and anxiety disorders, *J Psychopharmacol* (1998) **12**:161–7.

27. Glue P, White E, Wilson S, Ball D, Nutt DJ, The pharmacology of saccadic eye movements (2): effects of the α-2-adrenoceptor ligands idazoxan and clonidine, *Psychopharmacology* (1991) **105**:368–73.

28. Abelson JL, Glitz D, Cameron OG, et al, Blunted growth hormone response to clonidine in patients with generalized anxiety disorder, *Arch Gen Psychiatry* (1991); **48**: 157–62

29. Nutt DJ, Altered central alpha-2-adrenoceptor sensitivity in panic disorder. *Arch Gen Psychiatry* (1989) **46**:165–9.

30. Schittecatte M, Garcia-Valentin J, Charles G, et al, Efficacy of the "clonidine REM suppression test (CREST)" to separate patients with major depres-

sion from controls: a comparison with currently proposed biological markers of depression, *J Affect Disord* (1995) **33**:151–7.

31. El-Khayat R, Baldwin DS, Antipsychotic drugs for non-psychotic patients: assessment of the benefit/risk ratio in generalized anxiety disorder, *J Psychopharmacol* (1998) **12**:323–9

32. Schneier FR, Liebowitz MR, Abi-Dargham A, Zea-Ponce Y, Lin S-H, Laruelle M, Low dopamine D2 receptor binding potential in social phobia, *Am J Psych* (2000) **157**:457–9.

33. Tiihonen J, Kuikka J, Bergström K, et al, Dopamine re-uptake site densities in patients with social phobia. *Am J Psychiatry* (1997) **154**:239–42.

34. Malizia AL, Nutt DJ, Brain mechanisms and circuits in panic disorder. In: *Panic Disorder: Clinical Diagnosis, Management and Mechanisms,* eds: Nutt DJ, Ballenger JC, Lépine JP (Martin Dunitz Publishers, London 1998):55–77.

35. Nutt DJ, The pharmacology of human anxiety, *Pharmacol Ther* (1990) **47**:233–66.

36. Verburg K, Perna G, Griez EJL, A case study of the 35% CO_2 challenge. In: Griez EJL, Faravelli C, Nutt D, Zohar J, *Anxiety Disorders – An Introduction to Clinical Management and Research.* (John Wiley, Chichester, 2001) 341–57.

37. Argyropoulos SV, Bailey JE, Hood SD, Kendrick AH, Rich AS, Laszlo G, Nash JR, Lightman SL, Nutt, DJ, Inhalation of 35% CO_2 results in activation of the HPA axis in healthy volunteers, *Psychoneuroendocrinology*, in press.

38. Woods SW, Charney DS, Goodman WK, Heninger GR, Carbon dioxide-induced anxiety: Behavioral, physiologic and biochemical effects of carbon dioxide in patients with panic disorder and healthy subjects, *Arch Gen Psychiatry* (1988) **45**:43–52.

39. Bailey JE, Nash J, Kendrick A, Argyropoulos S, Nutt DJ, Psychological and psychomotor effects of inhaling 7.5% CO_2 for 20 minutes *J Psychopharmacol* (2001) **15**(3): A23.

6

Gene–environment Interactions in Generalized Anxiety Disorder

Klaus-Peter Lesch

Introduction

Although serotonergic and GABAergic dysfunction is likely to occur in generalized anxiety disorder (GAD), etiopathogenetic mechanisms continue to be inadequately understood at the neuronal and molecular level (see also Chapter 5). Functional imaging studies have revealed enhanced cortical activity and decreased basal ganglia activity in patients with GAD, which reverses with treatment. J.A. Gray's model[1] of behavioral inhibition, in which the septohippocampal system acts by assessing stimuli for the presence of threat or danger and, when that is detected, activates the behavioral-inhibition circuit, provides a neuroanatomic model that has been expanded by preclinical research.

A large body of evidence from family, twin, and adoptee studies has been accrued that a complex genetic component is involved in the vulnerability to anxiety disorders. While genetic research has typically focused either on anxiety-related traits or on anxiety disorders, with few investigations evaluating the genetic

and environmental relationship between the two, it is crucial to answer the question of whether a certain quantitative trait etiopathogenetically influences the disorder or whether the trait is a syndromal dimension of the disorder. This concept also supports the hypothesis that a genetic predisposition, coupled with early stress, in critical stages of development may result in a phenotype that is neurobiologically vulnerable to stress and may lower an individual's threshold for developing anxiety (or depression) on additional stress exposure.

A complementary approach to genetic studies of anxiety and related disorders involves investigation of genes (i.e. construction of transcriptome maps) and their protein products (i.e. application of proteomics) implicated in the brain neurocircuitry of anxiety in animal models. Based on an increasing body of evidence that genetically driven variability of expression and function of proteins that regulate the function of brain neurotransmitter systems (e.g. receptors, ion channels, transporters, and enzymes), is associated with complex behavioral traits, research is also giving emphasis to the molecular basis of anxiety-related behaviors in rodents and, increasingly, non-human primates.

Conditioning of fear and anxiety involves pathways transmitting information to and from the amygdala to various neural networks that control the expression of aggressive or defensive reactions, including behavioral, autonomic nervous system, and stress hormone responses (Figure 6.1).[2] While pathways from the thalamus and cortex (sensory and prefrontal) project to the amygdala, inputs are processed within intra-amygdaloid circuitries and outputs are directed to the hippocampus, brain stem, hypothalamus, and other regions.

Thus, the amygdala-associated neural network seems to be critical to integration of the 'fight or flight' response. In line with this notion it has recently been shown in rhesus monkeys that the amygdala mediates acute fear but not the behavioral and physiological components of anxious temperament.[3] Identification of molecular components of neural circuits involved in fear and anxiety is currently leading to new candidate genes of presumed pathophysiologic pathways, in addition to candidates that are generally derived from hypothesized pathogenetic mechanisms of the disorder or from clinical observations of therapeutic response.

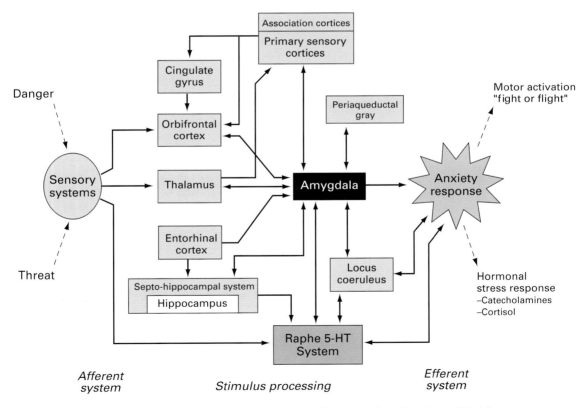

Figure 6.1 Serotonin and the functional neuroanatomy of fear and anxiety (modified from Charney and Deutch[55])

This chapter appraises fundamental aspects of the genetic component of anxiety-related traits with special emphasis on GAD. Pertinent concepts and methods in the search for candidate genes for anxiety and for the development of mouse models of human anxiety will also be discussed.

Anxiety-related traits

The dimensional structure of neuroticism or the anxiety-related cluster comprising fearfulness, emotional instability, and stress reactivity has been delineated by systematic research. Individual differences in anxiety-related traits, and the ultimate behavioral consequences of the 'fight or flight' response, are relatively enduring, continuously distributed, as well as substantially heritable, although they seem to result from additive or nonadditive interaction of genetic variations with environmental influences. While studies of the patterns of inheritance indicate that anxiety-related traits are likely to be influenced by a considerable number of genes, making them polygenic or quantitative traits, the studies likewise stress the significance of environmental factors. However, the relative influence of genetic and environmental factors on temperamental and behavioral differences is controversial and the complexities of gene–gene and gene–environment interactions are not well understood.

'Fight or flight' responses, which are the consequence of predominance of either aggressiveness and hostility or fearfulness and anxiety, seem to delineate a biologically based model of dispositions to both normal and pathological functioning, with a continuum of genetic risk underlying the behavioral dimensions that extend from normal to deviant. Thus, the analysis of the genetic component of anxiety-related behavior is both conceptually and methodologically quite demanding, so that consistent findings remain rare. The documented heterogeneity of both genetic and environmental determinants suggests the futility of searching for unitary causes. This vista has therefore increasingly encouraged the pursuit of dimensional and quantitative approaches to the genetics of anxiety-related traits, in addition to the classical strategy of studying individuals with anxiety disorders defined by consensus.

While quantitative genetics has focused on complex, quantitatively distributed traits and their origins in naturally occurring variation caused by multiple genetic and environmental factors, molecular genetics has begun to identify specific genes for quantitative traits, called quantitative trait loci (QTLs).[4] This perspective suggests that it may be less difficult to identify genes for psychopathology by searching for genes influencing personality, and that complex traits are not attributable to single genes necessary or sufficient to cause a disorder. The QTL concept thus implies that there may not be genes for psychiatric disorders, just genes for behavioral dimensions.

Because the power of linkage analysis to detect small gene effects is quite limited, at least with realistic samples, QTL research in humans has relied on association analysis using DNA variants in or near candidate genes that are functional. Gene variants with a significant impact on the functionality of components of brain neurotransmission, such as the serotonin (5HT) system, are a rational beginning. Based on converging lines of evidence that the 5HT and serotonergic gene expression are involved in a myriad of processes during brain development as well as synaptic plasticity in adulthood, temperamental predispositions and behavior are likely to be influenced by genetically driven variability of 5HT function. Consequently, the contribution of a polymorphism in the 5′-flanking regulatory region of the 5HT transporter gene (5HTTLPR) to individual phenotypic differences in anxiety-related traits was explored in independent population- and family-based genetic studies.[5,6] Evidence is accumulating that 5HT transporter gene variability results in allelic variation of 5HT transporter expression and function, which is associated with personality traits of negative emotionality including anxiety, depression, and aggressiveness (neuroticism and agreeableness).

The effect sizes for the 5HTTLPR-personality associations indicate that this polymorphism has a moderate influence on these behavioral predispositions that corresponds to less than 5% of the total variance, based on estimates from twin studies using these and related measures which have consistently demonstrated that genetic factors contribute 40–60% of the variance in neuroticism and other related personality traits. The associations represent only a modest share of the genetic contribution to anxiety-related traits. Additive contributions of comparable size or epistatic interaction have, in fact, been found

in studies of other quantitative traits. Thus, the results are consistent with the view that the influence of a single, common polymorphism on continuously distributed traits is likely to be modest, if not minimal.

A growing body of evidence implicates personality traits, such as neuroticism or negative emotionality, in the comorbidity of affective spectrum disorders[7,8] (Figure 6.2). Separation of mental illness from personality disorders in current consensual diagnostic systems remarkably enhanced interest in the link between temperament, personality, and psychiatric disorders as well as the impact of this interrelationship on the heterogeneity within diagnostic entities, prediction of long-term course, and treatment response.[9] Based on multivariate genetic analyses of comorbidity, generalized anxiety disorder and major depression have common genetic origins and the phenotypic differences between anxiety and depression are dependent upon the environment.[10] Moreover, indexed by the personality scale of neuroticism, general vulnerability overlaps genetically to a substantial extent with both anxiety and depression. These

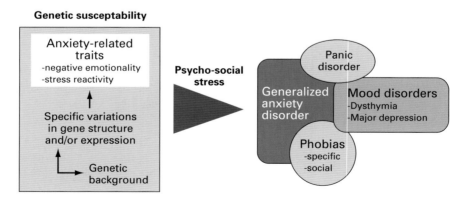

Figure 6.2 Structural relationship of the dimensions comprising anxiety-related personality traits and various anxiety and mood disorders (adapted from Lesch[23]). Anxiety-related personality traits and generalized anxiety disorder-associated negative affect and worry are conceptualized as dispositional traits common to both anxiety and mood disorders including depression.

results predicted that when a QTL, such as the 5HTTLPR, is found for neuroticism, the same QTL should be associated with symptoms of anxiety and depression. Anxiety and mood disorders are therefore likely to represent the extreme end of variation in negative emotionality.[4] The genetic factor contributing to the extreme ends of dimensions of variation commonly recognized as a disorder may be quantitatively, not qualitatively, different from the rest of the distribution. This has important implications for identifying genes for complex traits related to a distinct disorder. An association of the 5HTTLPR and affective illness including unipolar depression and bipolar disorder has been reported by several but not all investigators.[11] Reasons for these conflicting results are manifold and several caveats have to be kept in mind. Particularly misleading are both false-positive and false-negative findings due to population stratification as well as gene–gene and gene–environment interactions. False-negative association studies impede further research, as they are unlikely to be replicated, whereas truly negative studies are under-represented due to publication bias, an error with declining impact, since this problem is increasingly acknowledged by scientists, reviewers, and editors. Because QTL loci require impractically large sets of sib pairs to gain sufficient statistical power in linkage analyses, candidate gene studies are more feasible despite these limitations.

Generalized anxiety disorder

GAD is defined by excessive and uncontrollable worry about a number of life events or activities for least 6 months, accompanied by at least 3 of 6 associated symptoms of negative affect or tension, such as restlessness, fatigue, concentration difficulties, irritability, muscle tension, sleep disturbance. Studies of the lifetime prevalence for GAD in the general population have provided estimates ranging from 1.6 to 5.1% and indicated a 2:1 female-to-male preponderance.[12,13] Relative to other anxiety and mood disorders, GAD is more likely to show a gradual onset and/or life-long history of symptoms. While early ages of onset are common, the syndrome itself may emerge only later in life and a considerable number of patients with GAD report an onset in adulthood that is usually in response to psychosocial stress. Research has consistently shown that GAD is associated with high comorbidity rates for other disorders, including panic anxiety, social phobia, specific phobia, dysthymia, and major depression (Figure 6.2).[14,15] Moreover, patients with GAD frequently undergo treatment for stress-associated physical conditions (e.g. chronic pain syndromes). Studies have begun to address the structural relationship of the dimensions comprising various anxiety disorders and there is an increasing body of evidence that GAD-associated negative affect and worry are dispositional traits common to both anxiety and depression (Figure 6.1). GAD may therefore be conceptionalized as a trait or vulnerability dimension predisposing to other disorders, and etiological models of GAD integrate both psychosocial and biological factors.[16]

Twin- and family-based studies indicate a clear genetic influence in GAD with a heritability of approximately 15–40%.[17,18] GAD-associated genetic factors are completely shared with depression, while environmental determinants seem to be distinct.[10,15] This notion is consistent with recent models of emotional disorders which view anxiety and mood disorders as sharing common vulnerabilities but differing on dimensions including, for instance, focus of attention or psychosocial liability.[19] See Chapter 1 for a different view of this data.

Familial patterns of aggregation also suggest that GAD, panic disorder, agoraphobia, and depression may co-occur, but it is still a matter of considerable debate whether they have related or different genetic etiologies. Despite this controversy, the results of several genomic scans for susceptibility loci for panic disorder as well as association studies of candidate genes in patients with panic disorder should be mentioned here, because these loci and genes may also influence the risk for GAD. Three complete genome-wide linkage scans for panic disorder liability genes have recently been published.[20,21,22] Linkage analyses are based on the identification of large, densely affected families so that the inheritance patterns of known sections of DNA, such as polymorphic repetitive elements, can be compared to the family's transmission of the disorder. Linkage of a particular allele to the presence or absence of a phenotype which breeds true allows researchers to define and narrow down the location of the suspect gene. Although none of the findings based on lod scores or the proportion of allele sharing reached a level of statistical confidence according to the stringent Lander-Kruglyak criteria, a region suggestive of a susceptibility locus for panic disorder on chromosome 7p15 was independently identified in both studies. Crowe and associates[21] detected the highest lod score of 2.23 at the D7S2846 locus, located at 57.8 cM on chromosome 7, in a region that lies within 15 cM from the D7S435 locus reported by Knowles et al.[20] Gelernter and coworkers[22] reported two genomic loci in panic disorder meeting criteria for suggestive linkage, one is located on chromosome 1 (lod score, 2.04), the other on chromosome 11p with a lod score of 2.01. For agoraphobia, potential linkage was detected on chromosome 3 which was accounted for primarily by a single family, suggesting that panic disorder and agoraphobia may share some, but not all, of their susceptibility loci. Some of the conflicting results of past linkage analyses may be ascribed to methodological differences in family ascertainment, phenotype definition, diagnostic assessment, and data analysis. Even more likely, they may represent true etiologic differences due to locus heterogeneity. Susceptibility to panic disorder may thus be influenced either by an incompletely penetrant major gene in some families or by multiple genes of weak and varying effect in others.

Since evidence for a genetic component in anxiety disorder in general and panic disorder/agoraphobia in particular is compelling, a small number of putative risk genes have been assessed in association studies. Candidate genes were selected in consideration of components of neurotransmitter systems involved in anxiogenic responses or therapeutic action of anxiolytic drugs. Studies of genetic association compare the frequency of a particular polymorphism in patients with controls, or compare scores on a continuous measure for two groups with a genetic marker of interest. Because quantitative traits are influenced by multiple genes of varying effect size and by environmental factors, QTLs for complex traits such as anxiety are likely to be of very modest, if not minimal, effect size and thus account for only a small proportion of the variance in the population.

Although it may be hypothesized that enhanced serotonergic neurotransmission in panic disorder is due to decreased 5HT uptake, no association with 5HTTLPR-dependent variation in 5HT transporter expression and panic disorder was detected in different populations.[23] These negative findings are compatible with the assumption that additional or alternative cellular pathways and neural circuits are involved in anxiety. Monoamine oxidase A (MAOA), an enzyme involved in the degradation of 5HT and norepinephrine and thus positioned at the crossroads of two monoaminergic systems, is another plausible candidate gene. Assessment of a MAOA gene-linked polymorphic region (MAOALPR), which shows allele-dependent transcriptional efficiency, for association with panic disorder in two independent samples showed that high activity alleles were significantly more frequent in female patients than in females of the corresponding control populations.[24] The co-occurrence of panic and phobic disorders with joint laxity recently facilitated the identification of an interstitial duplication of human chromosome 15q24–26, named DUP25.[25] Mosaicism, different forms of DUP25 within the same family, and absence of segregation of 15q24–26 markers with DUP25 and psychiatric phenotypes suggest a non-Mendelian mechanism of disease-causing mutation. Finally, no significant associations between panic disorder and alleles of the GABA-A, GABA-B, dopamine D2 and D4, dopamine transporter, cholecystokinin B or the adenosine A1 and A2a receptor genes have been detected.[23]

Animal models

Quantitative genetic research on animal models consists primarily of inbred strain and selection studies. While comparisons between different inbred strains of mice expose remarkable differences in measures of anxiety-related behavior, differences within strains can be attributed to environmental influences. Inbred and recombinant inbred strain studies are highly efficient in dissecting genetic influences, for investigating interactions between genotype and environment, and for testing the disposition–stress model.

Selective breeding of mice for many generations produces differences between high and low anxiety lines that steadily increase each generation. Selection studies of behavioral traits strongly suggest a genetic influence and that many genes contribute to variation in behavior. Mice strains that have been selectively bred to display a phenotype of interest are currently being used to identify genetic loci that contribute to behavioral traits including fearfulness and emotionality.[26,27] However, linkage analyses provide only a rough chromosomal localization, whereas the next step, identifying the relevant genes by positional cloning, remains a challenging task. Since mice and humans share many orthologous genes mapped to synthenic chromosomal regions, it is conceivable that individual genes identified for one or more types of murine anxiety-related behavior may be developed as animal models for human anxiety. Following chromosomal mapping of polymorphic genes and evaluation of gene function using knock-out mutants, behavioral parameters, including the type of anxiety, measure of anxiety, test situation and opponent type are investigated. Thus, the combination of elaborate genetic and behavioral analyses results in the identification of many genes with effects on variation and development of murine anxiety-related behavior and, ultimately, mouse QTL research is likely to generate candidate QTL for human anxiety disorders.

Recent advances in gene targeting (constitutive or conditional knockout and knockin techniques) are increasingly impacting upon our understanding of the neurobiologic basis of anxiety-related behavior in mice. However, the majority of neural substrates and circuitries that regulate emotional processes or cause anxiety disorders remain remarkably elusive. Among the reasons for the lack of progress are several conceptional deficiencies regarding the psychobiology of fear and anxiety, which make it difficult to develop and validate reliable models. The clinical presentation of anxiety disorders and the lack of consensus on clinical categories further complicates the development of mouse models for specific anxiety disorders. The dilemma that no single paradigm mimics the diagnostic entities or treatment response of anxiety disorders may reflect the inadequacy of classification rather than failure to develop valid mouse models.

Various approaches have been employed to study anxiety-related traits in mice and the majority postulate that aversive stimuli, such as novelty or potentially harmful environments induce a central state of fear and defensive reactions, which can be assessed and quantified through physiologic and behavioral paradigms.[28] While substantial similarities between human and murine avoidance, defense or escape response exist, it remains obscure whether mice also experience subjective anxiety and associated cognitive processes similar to humans or whether defense responses represent pathological forms of anxiety in humans. However, it seems a reasonable assumption that pathological anxiety may reflect an inappropriate activation of normally adaptive, evolutionarily conserved defense reactions. It should therefore be practicable to elucidate both physiologic and pathologic anxiety by studying avoidant and defensive behavior in mice using a broad range of anxiety models to ensure comprehensive characterization of the behavioral phenotype.

The design of a mouse model partially or completely lacking a gene-of-interest during all stages of development (constitutive knockout) is among the prime strategies directed at elucidating the role of genetic factors in fear and anxiety. Following the landmark studies by Mohler and coworkers[29] who generated mice lacking the γ_2 subunit of the GABA-A (gamma-aminobutyric acid type A) receptor, a notable body of evidence has been accumulated that GABA-A function is compromised in anxiety disorders (for review see Nutt and Malizia[30]). Heterozygous GABA-A γ_2 subunit knockout mice are less sensitive to benzodiazepines, display hypervigilance and anxiety, and show decreases in ligand binding throughout the brain. These mice may represent a genetically defined model of trait anxiety that closely mimics the pharmacological, morphological, and behavioral phenotype of human anxiety disorders. Various other types of GABA-A subunits, including α_1, α_2, α_3, and β_3, have been genetically altered in mice by introducing a defined mutation (constitutive knockin).[31,32] While mice with a mutated α_1 subtype gene are insensitive to the sedative actions of benzodiazepines but are still responsive to GABA, the anxiolytic effect is lost if the α_2 but not the α_3 subtype is modified. The localization of the γ_2 subtype in the limbic system further supports a role of this neurocircuit in anxiety.

A possible role for the $5HT_{1A}$ receptor in the modulation of anxiety (and depression) as well as in the mode of action of anxiolytic and antidepressant drugs has been suspected for many years. $5HT_{1A}$ receptors operate both as somatodendritic autoreceptors and as postsynaptic receptors. Somatodendritic $5HT_{1A}$ autoreceptors are predominantly located on 5HT neurons and dendrites in the midbrain raphe complex and their activation by 5HT or $5HT_{1A}$ agonists decreases the firing rate of serotonergic neurons and subsequently reduces the release of 5HT from nerve terminals. Postsynaptic $5HT_{1A}$ receptors are widely distributed in brain regions that receive serotonergic input, notably in the cortex, hippocampus, and hypothalamus. Their activation results in neuronal inhibition, the consequences of which are not well understood, and in physiological responses that depend upon the function of the target cells (e.g. activation of the hypothalamic pituitary adrenocortical system). Recently, several papers reported the generation of mice with a targeted inactivation of the $5HT_{1A}$ receptor.[33,34,35]

Mice with a targeted inactivation of the $5HT_{1A}$ receptor consistently display a spontaneous phenotype that is associated with a gender-modulated and gene/dose-dependent increase of anxiety-related behaviors. With the exception of an enhanced sensitivity of terminal $5HT_{1B}$ receptors and downregulation of GABA-A receptors,[36] no major neuroadaptational changes were detected. Noteworthy is that this behavioral phenotype was observed in animals of different backgrounds into which the mutation had been bred, validating the assumption that this behavior is an authentic consequence of reduced or absent $5HT_{1A}$ receptors. While all research groups used Open Field exploratory behavior as a model for assessing anxiety, two groups confirmed that $5HT_{1A}$ knockout mice had increased anxiety by using other models, the Elevated Zero Maze or Elevated Plus Maze test. These ethologically based conflict models test fear and anxiety-related behaviors based on the natural tendencies for rodents to prefer enclosed, dark spaces versus their interest in exploring novel environments.

Activation of presynaptic $5HT_{1A}$ receptors provides the brain with an autoinhibitory feedback system controlling 5HT neurotransmission. Thus, enhanced anxiety-related behavior most likely represents a consequence of increased terminal 5HT availability resulting from the lack of or reduction in presynaptic somatodendritic $5HT_{1A}$ autoreceptor negative feedback function. Indirect evidence for increased presynaptic serotonergic activity is provided by the compensatory upregulation of terminal $5HT_{1B}$ receptors. This mechanism is also consistent with recent theoretical models of fear and anxiety that are primarily based upon pharmacologically derived data. The cumulative reduction in serotonergic impulse flow to septohippocampal and other limbic and cortical areas involved in the control of anxiety is believed to explain the anxiolytic effects of ligands with selective affinity for the $5HT_{1A}$ receptor in some animal models of anxiety-related behavior. This notion is based, in part, on evidence that $5HT_{1A}$ agonists and antagonists have anxiolytic or anxiogenic effects, respectively. However, to complicate matters further, 8-OH-DPAT has anxiolytic effects when injected in the raphe nucleus, whereas it is anxiogenic when applied to the hippocampus. Thus, stimulation of postsynaptic $5HT_{1A}$ receptors has been proposed to elicit anxiogenic effects, while activation of $5HT_{1A}$ autoreceptors is thought to induce anxiolytic effects via suppression of serotonergic neuronal firing resulting in attenuated 5HT release in limbic terminal fields.

Excess serotonergic neurotransmission may also be implicated in increased anxiety-related behaviors recently found in 5HT transporter-deficient mice.[37] These findings are consistent with other evidence suggesting that increased 5HT availability may contribute to increased anxiety in rodents, and the studies reporting that anxiety-related traits in humans are associated with allelic variation of 5HT transporter function[3]. Mice with a disrupted 5HT transporter gene have been suggested as an alternative model to pharmacological studies of SSRI-evoked antidepressant and anxiolytic mechanisms to assess the hypothesized association between 5HT uptake function and $5HT_{1A}$ receptor desensitization.[38] Excess serotonergic neurotransmission in mice lacking 5HT transport results in desensitized and, unlike observations following SSRI administration, downregulated $5HT_{1A}$ receptors in the midbrain raphe complex but not in the hippocampus[39] and is suspected to play a role in the increased anxiety-related behaviors in these mice using the Light-Dark and Elevated Zero Maze paradigms. In contrast to $5HT_{1A}$-deficient mice, anxiety-related behavior is more pronounced in female 5HT transporter null mutants. However, anxiety-related behavior can be reversed by anxiolytics of the benzodiazepine type in both knockout strains.

Morphological analyses of cortical and subcortical structures where 5HT has been suggested to act as a differentiation signal in cortical development revealed an impact of 5HT transporter inactivation on the formation and plasticity of brain structures. Inactivation of the 5HT transporter gene profoundly disturbs formation of the somatosensory cortex (SSC) with altered cytoarchitecture of cortical layer IV, the layer that contains synapses between thalamocortical terminals and their postsynaptic target neurons.[40] These findings demonstrate that excessive amounts of extracellular 5HT are damaging to SSC development and suggest that transient 5HT transporter expression in thalamocortical neurons is responsible for barrel patterns in neonatal rodents, and its permissive action is required for barrel pattern formation, presumably by maintaining extracellular 5HT concentrations below a critical threshold.[41] Since the gene-dose dependent reduction in 5HT transporter availability in heterozygous mice that leads

to a modest delay in 5HT uptake but distinctive irregularities in barrel and septum shape is similar to those reported in humans carrying a low activity allele of the 5HTTLPR, it may be speculated that allelic variation in 5HT transporter function also affects the human brain during development with due consequences for personality, disease liability, and therapeutic response.

The evidence that changes in 5HT system homeostasis exert long-term effects on cortical development and adult brain plasticity may be an important step forward in establishing the psychobiological groundwork for a neurodevelopmental hypothesis of neuroticism, negative emotionality, and anxiety disorders. Although there is converging evidence that serotonergic dysfunction contributes to anxiety-related behavior, the precise mechanism that renders $5HT_{1A}$ receptor and 5HT transporter-deficient mice more anxious remains to be elucidated. While increased 5HT availability and activation of other serotonergic receptor subtypes that have been shown to mediate anxiety (e.g. $5HT_{2C}$ receptor) may contribute to increased anxiety in the rodent model, multiple downstream cellular pathways or neurocircuits, including noradrenergic, GABAergic, glutamatergic, and peptidergic transmission, as suggested by overexpression or targeted inactivation of critical genes within these systems, have been implicated to participate in the processing of this complex behavioral trait. Recent work has therefore been focused on a large number of genes that have known relevance in the neurocircuitries of fear and anxiety, although the knockout of some genes that appear not to be directly involved in anxiety may also lead to an anxiety-related phenotype (Figure 6.3). For a review see Lesch[23] and references therein.

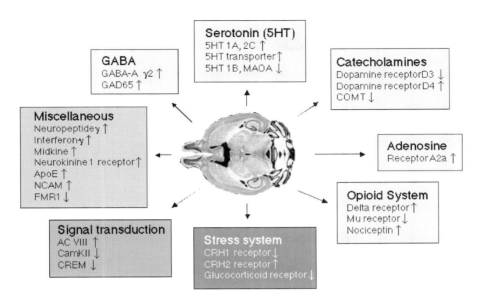

Figure 6.3 Knockout mice displaying an anxiety-related phenotype and behavior.[23] GABA, γ-amino butyric acid; GAD65, 65-kDa isoform of glutamic acid decarboxylase; MAOA, monoamine oxidase A; COMT, catechol-O-methyltransferase; AC VIII, adenylyl cyclase type VIII; CamKII, calcium–calmodulin kinase II; CRH corticotropin-releasing hormone; CREM, cAMP-responsive element modulator; ApoE, apolipoprotein E; NCAM, neural cell adhesion molecule; FMR1, Fragile X syndrome gene; ↑/↓, increase/decrease in anxiety-related behavior.

Gene–environment interactions

In the evaluation of complex genetic effects it is essential to control for environmental factors. The relationship between emotional reactions to stress (emotionality) and behavioral disorders is also central to the disposition–stress model of syndromal dimensions of anxiety disorders, in which the expression of genetic vulnerability is triggered by stress.[4,42] In line with this notion a twin study suggests that genetic liability to depression interacts with the presence of stressful life events in producing the outcome of anxiety and depression.[43] Additional, although preliminary, evidence comes from studies of rhesus macaques, a higher non-human primate species that like humans carries the 5HT transporter gene-associated polymorphism (rh5HTTLPR).

Previous work in rhesus monkeys has shown that early adverse experiences have long-term consequences for the functioning of the central 5HT system, as indicated by robustly lowered CSF 5HIAA levels as well as anxiety and depression-related behavior, in monkeys deprived of their parents at birth and raised only with peers.[44,45] Accumulating evidence demonstrates the complex interplay between individual differences in the central 5HT system and social success. In monkeys, lowered 5HT functioning, as indicated by decreased CSF 5HIAA levels, is associated with lower rank within a social group, less competent social behavior, and greater impulsive aggression. Association between central 5HT turnover and rh5HTTLPR genotype was tested in rhesus monkeys with well-characterized environmental histories.[46] The monkeys' rearing fell into one of the following categories: mother-reared, either reared with the biological mother or cross-fostered; or peer-reared, either with a peer group of 3–4 monkeys or with an inanimate surrogate and daily contact with a playgroup of peers. Peer-reared monkeys were separated from their mothers, placed in the nursery at birth, and given access to peers at 30 days of age either continuously or during daily play sessions. Mother-reared and cross-fostered monkeys remained with the mother, typically within a social group. At roughly 7 months of age, mother-reared monkeys were weaned and placed together with their peer-reared cohort in large, mixed-gender social groups.

Since the monkey population comprised two groups that received dramatically different social and rearing experience early in life, the interactive effects of environmental experience and the rh5HTTLPR on cisternal CSF 5HIAA levels and 5HT-related behavior were assessed. CSF 5HIAA concentrations were significantly influenced by genotype for peer-reared, but not for mother-reared, subjects. Peer-reared rhesus monkeys with the low-activity rh5HTTLPR short allele had significantly lower concentrations of CSF 5HIAA than their homozygous long/long counterparts. Low 5HT turnover in monkeys with the short allele is congruent with in vitro studies that show reduced binding and transcriptional efficiency of the 5HT transporter gene associated with the short 5HTTLPR allele in humans.[5] This suggests that the rh5HTTLPR genotype is predictive of CSF 5HIAA concentrations, but that early experiences make unique contributions to variation in later 5HT functioning. This finding is the first to provide evidence of an environment-dependent association between a polymorphism in the 5HT transporter gene and a direct measure of 5HT functioning, cisternal CSF 5HIAA concentration, thus revealing an interaction between rearing environment and rhHTTLPR genotype. Similar to the 5HTTLPR's influence on anxiety-related traits in humans, however, the effect size is small, with 4.7% of variance in CSF 5HIAA accounted for by the rh5HTTLPR–rearing environment interaction.

Recent studies have also focused on the neonatal period, a time in early development when environmental influences are minimal and least likely to confound associations between temperament and genes. In this context the term temperament is used to refer to the psychological qualities of infants that display considerable variation and have a relatively, but not indefinitely, stable biological basis in the indivdual's genotype, even though different phenotypes may emerge as the child grows.[47,48] In order to facilitate investigation of the contribution of genotype and early rearing environment to the development of behavioral traits, complementary approaches have recently been applied to nonhuman primate behavioral genetics. Rhesus macaque infants heterozygous for the short and long variant of the rhHTTLPR displayed higher behavioral stress-reactivity compared with infants homozygous for the long variant of the allele.[49,50] Mother-reared and peer-reared monkeys were assessed on days 7, 14, 21, and 30 of life, on a standardized primate neurobehavioral test designed to measure orienting, motor maturity, reflex functioning, and temperament. Main effects of genotype, and, in some cases, interactions between rearing condition and genotype, were demonstrated for items indicative of orienting, attention, and temperament. In general, rhHTTLPR heterozygote animals demonstrated diminished orientation, lower attentional capabilities, and increased affective responding relative to long/long homozygotes. However, the genotype effects were more pronounced for animals raised in the neonatal nursery than for animals reared by their mothers. These results demonstrate the contributions of rearing environment and genetic background, and their interaction, in a non-human primate model of behavioral development.

Taken together, these findings provide evidence of an environment-dependent association between allelic variation of 5HT transporter expression and central 5HT function, and illustrate the possibility that specific genetic factors play a role in social competence and related traits. The objective of further studies will be the elucidation of the relationship between the genotypes and sociality in monkeys as this behavior is expressed with characteristic individual differences both in daily life and in response to challenge. Because rhesus monkeys exhibit temperamental and behavioral traits that parallel anxiety, depression, and aggression-related personality dimensions associated in humans with the low-activity 5HTTLPR variant, it may be possible to search for evolutionary continuity in this genetic mechanism for individual differences.

The biobehavioral results of deleterious early experiences of social separation are consistent with the notion that the 5HTTLPR may influence the risk for anxiety spectrum disorders. Evolutionary preservation of two prevalent 5HTTLPR variants and the resulting allelic variation in 5HT transporter expression may be part of the genetic mechanism resulting in the emergence of temperamental traits that facilitate adaptive functioning in the complex social worlds most primates inhabit. The uniqueness of the 5HTTLPR among humans and simian non-human primates, but not among prosimians or other mammals, along with the role 5HT plays in complex primate sociality, form the basis for the hypothesized relationship between the 5HT transporter function and personality traits that mediate individual differences in social behavior. Non-human primate studies may therefore be useful to help identify environmental factors that either compound the vulnerability conferred by a particular genetic makeup or, conversely, act to improve the behavioral outcome associated with that genotype.

Conclusions

Progress in the genetics of anxiety-related traits and behavior is currently expedited by integration of neuroscience and genetics. More functionally relevant polymorphisms in genes within a single neurotransmitter system, or in genes which comprise a developmental and functional unit in their concerted actions, need to be identified and investigated. Not only will DNA variants in coding and regulatory regions of genes be useful for systematic genome scans for identifying genes associated with personality and behavior, they will also make it possible to study integrated systems of gene pathways as an important step on the route to behavioral genomics. Although progress has been made in understanding the diversity of the human genome, such as the frequency, distribution, and type of genetic variation that exists, the feasibility of applying this information to uncover useful genomic markers for behavioral traits remains uncertain. Based on the first draft sequence of the human genome, several million single nucleotide polymorphisms (SNPs) in addition to microdeletions (or insertions), and polymorphic simple sequence repeats (SSRs) of 2 to 50+ nucleotides in length have been identified in the human genome, yet no more than roughly 30,000–60,000 common polymorphisms are located in coding and regulatory regions of genes which are the ultimate causes of the heritability of complex traits.[51,52]

Rarely addressed are issues related to the reality of using SNPs to uncover markers for behavioral traits and disorders as well as treatment response, such as population and patient sample size, SNP density and genome coverage, SNP functionality, and data interpretation that will be important for determining the suitability of genomic information. Success will depend on the availability of SNPs in the coding or regulatory regions (cSNPs or rSNPs, respectively) of a large number of candidate genes as well as knowledge of the average extent of linkage disequilibrium between SNPs, the development of high-throughput technologies for genotyping SNPs, identification of protein-altering SNPs by DNA and protein microarray-assisted expression analysis, and collection of DNA from well-assessed cohorts. As more and more appreciation of the potential for polymorphisms in gene regulatory regions to impact gene expression is gained, knowledge of novel functional variants is likely to emerge.

Anxiety and related traits are generated by a complex interaction of environmental and experiental factors with a number of genes and their products. Even pivotal regulatory proteins of cellular pathways and neurocircuits are most likely to have only a very modest, if not minimal, impact, while noise from nongenetic mechanisms obstructs identification of relevant gene variants. Investigation of gene–environment interactions in humans and non-human primates as well as gene inactiva-

tion studies in mice further intensify the identification of genes that are essential for development and adult plasticity of the brain related to anxiety.

Association studies in large cohorts are required to elucidate complex epistatic and epigenetic interactions of multiple loci with the environment. In order to minimize the risk of population stratification bias, rigorous methods of 'genomic control' have been designed. These statistical strategies are based on the assessment of 60 SNPs or genotypes of 100 unlinked microsatellite markers spread throughout the genome to adjust the significance level of a candidate gene polymorphism.[53,54] With recent advances in molecular genetics, the rate-limiting step in identifying candidate genes has nevertheless become the definition of phenotype.

Future research will take advantage of the completion of the sequencing of the human and mouse genomes coinciding with the revolution in bioinformatics. Integration of these emerging technologies for genetic analysis will provide the basis for gene identification and functional studies in GAD.

Summary

Genetic epidemiology has assembled convincing evidence that anxiety-related traits and generalized anxiety disorder (GAD) are influenced by genetic factors and that the genetic component is highly complex, polygenic, and epistatic. Because the mode of inheritance of GAD is complex, it has been concluded that multiple genes of modest effect, in interaction with each other and in conjunction with environmental events, produce vulnerability to the disorder. Investigation of gene–environment interactions in humans and non-human primates as well as gene inactivation studies in mice further intensify the identification of genes that are essential for development and plasticity of brain systems related to anxiety. Future research will take advantage of the completion of the sequencing of the human and mouse genome coinciding with the revolution in bioinformatics. Integration of these emerging technologies for genetic analysis will provide the basis for gene identification and functional studies in GAD.

References

1. Gray JA, *The Psychology of Fear and Stress* (Cambridge University Press, Cambridge, 1988).

2. Gorman JM, Kent JM, Sullivan GM, Coplan JD, Neuroanatomical hypothesis of panic disorder, revised, *Am J Psychiatry* (2000) **157**:493–505.

3. Kalin NH, Shelton SE, Davidson RJ, Kelley AE, The primate amygdala mediates acute fear but not the behavioral and physiological components of anxious temperament, *J Neurosci* (2001) **21**: 2067–74.

4. Eley TC, Plomin R, Genetic analyses of emotionality, *Curr Opin Neurobiol* (1997) **7**:279–84.

5. Lesch KP, Bengel D, Heils A, et al, Association of anxiety-related traits with a polymorphism in the serotonin transporter gene regulatory region, *Science* (1996) **274**:1527–31.

6. Lesch KP, Greenberg BD, Bennett A, Higley JD, Murphy DL, Serotonin transporter, personality, and behavior: toward dissection of gene-gene and gene-environment interaction. In *Molecular Genetics and the Human Personality*, Benjamin J, Ebstein R, Belmaker RH (eds), (Washington, DC: American Psychiatric Press, 2002).

7. Jardine R, Martin NG, Henderson AS, Genetic covariation between neuroticism and the symptoms of anxiety and depression, *Genet Epidemiol* (1984) **1**:89–107.

8. Kendler KS, Neale MC, Kessler RC, Heath AC, Eaves LJ, A longitudinal twin study of personality and major depression in women, *Arch Gen Psychiatry* (1993) **50**:853–62.

9. Mulder RT, Joyce PR, Cloninger CR, Temperament and early environment influence comorbidity and personality disorders in major depression, *Compr Psychiatry* (1994) **35**:225–33.

10. Kendler KS, Major depression and generalised anxiety disorder. Same genes, (partly) different environments—revisited, *Br J Psychiatry* (1996) **30**(Suppl) 68–75.

11. Lesch KP, Serotonin transporter: from genomics and knockouts to behavioral traits and psychiatric disorders. In *Molecular Genetics of Mental Disorders*, Briley M, Sulser F (eds), 221–67. (London: Martin Dunitz Publishers 2001a).

12. Torgersen S, Genetic factors in anxiety disorders, *Arch Gen Psychiatry* (1983) **40**:1085–9.

13. Lyons MJ, Huppert J, Toomey R, et al, Lifetime prevalence of mood and anxiety disorders in twin pairs discordant for schizophrenia, *Twin Res* (2000) **3**:28–32.

14. Skre I, Onstad S, Edvardsen J, Torgersen S, Kringlen E, A family study of anxiety disorders: familial transmission and relationship to mood disorder and psychoactive substance use disorder, *Acta Psychiatr Scand* (1994) **90**:366–74.

15. Roy MA, Neale MC, Pedersen NL, Mathe AA, Kendler KS, A twin study of generalized anxiety disorder and major depression, *Psychol Med* (1995) **25**:1037–49.

16. Silberg J, Rutter M, Neale M, Eaves L, Genetic moderation of environmental risk for depression and anxiety in adolescent girls, *Br J Psychiatry* (2001) **179**:116–21.

17. Scherrer JF, True WR, Xian H, et al, Evidence for genetic influences common and specific to symptoms of generalized anxiety and panic, *J Affect Disord* (2000) **57**:25–35.

18. Hettema JM, Prescott CA, Kendler KS, A population-based twin study of generalized anxiety disorder in men and women. *J Nerv Ment Dis* (2001) **189**:413–20.

19. Rijsdijk FV, Sham PC, Sterne A, et al, Life events and depression in a community sample of siblings, *Psychol Med* (2001) **31**:401–10.

20. Knowles JA, Fyer AJ, Vieland VJ, et al, Results of a genome-wide genetic screen for panic disorder, *Am J Med Genet* (1998) **81**:139–47.

21. Crowe RR, Goedken R, Samuelson S, et al, Genomewide survey of panic disorder, *Am J Med Genet* (2001) **105**:105–9.

22. Gelernter J, Bonvicini K, Page G, et al, Linkage genome scan for loci predisposing to panic disorder or agoraphobia, *Am J Med Genet* (2001) **105**: 548–57.

23. Lesch KP, Genetic dissection of anxiety and related disorders. In *Anxiety disorders*, Nutt D, Ballenger T (eds), (Oxford: Blackwell 2001b).

24. Deckert J, Catalano M, Syagailo YV, et al, Excess of high activity monoamine oxidase A gene promoter alleles in female patients with panic disorder, *Hum Mol Genet* (1999) **8**:621–4.

25. Gratacos M, Nadal M, Martin-Santos R, A polymorphic genomic duplication on human chromosome 15 is a susceptibility factor for panic and phobic disorders, *Cell* (2001) **106**:367–79.

26. Flint J, Corley R, DeFries JC, A simple genetic basis for a complex psychological trait in laboratory mice, *Science* (1995) **269**:1432–5.

27. Phillips TJ, Huson M, Gwiazdon C, Burkhart-Kasch S, Shen EH, Effects of acute and repeated ethanol exposures on the locomotor activity of BXD recombinant inbred mice, *Alcohol Clin Exp Res* (1995) **19**:269–78.

28. Crawley JN, Behavioral phenotyping of transgenic and knockout mice: experimental design and evaluation of general health, sensory functions, motor abilities, and specific behavioral tests, *Brain Res* (1999) **835**:18–26.

29. Crestani F, Lorez M, Baer K, et al, Decreased GABAA-receptor clustering results in enhanced anxiety and a bias for threat cues, *Nat Neurosci* (1999) **2**:833–9.

30. Nutt DJ, Malizia AL, New insights into the role of the GABA(A)-benzodiazepine receptor in psychiatric disorder, (2001) **179**:390–6.

31. Rudolph U, Crestani F, Benke D, et al, Benzodiazepine actions mediated by specific gamma-aminobutyric acid(A) receptor subtypes, *Nature* (1999) **401**:796–800.

32. Low K, Crestani F, Keist R, et al, Molecular and neuronal substrate for the selective attenuation of anxiety, *Science* (2000) **290**:131–4.

33. Heisler LK, Chu HM, Brennan TJ, Danao JA, Bajwa P, Parsons LH, Tecott LH, Elevated anxiety and antidepressant-like responses in serotonin 5-HT1A receptor mutant mice [see comments]. *Proc Natl Acad Sci U S A* (1998) **95**:15049–54.

34. Parks CL, Robinson PS, Sibille E, Shenk T, Toth M, Increased anxiety of mice lacking the serotonin1A receptor, *Proc Natl Acad Sci U S A* (1998) **95**:10734–9.

35. Ramboz S, Oosting R, Amara DA, et al, Serotonin receptor 1A knockout: an animal model of anxiety-related disorder [see comments]. *Proc Natl Acad Sci U S A* (1998) **95**:14476–81.

36. Sibille E, Pavlides C, Benke D, Toth M, Genetic inactivation of the serotonin(1A) receptor in mice results in downregulation of major GABA(A) receptor alpha subunits, reduction of GABA(A) receptor binding, and benzodiazepine-resistant anxiety, *J Neurosci* (2000) **20**:2758–65.

37. Wichems CH, Li Q, Holmes A, et al, Mechanisms mediating the increased anxiety-like behavior and excessive responses to stress in mice lacking the serotonin transporter, *Society of Neuroscience Abstract* (2000) **26**:400.

38. Bengel D, Murphy DL, Andrews AM, et al, Altered brain serotonin homeostasis and locomotor insensitivity to 3, 4-methylenedioxymethamphetamine ('Ecstasy') in serotonin transporter-deficient mice, *Mol Pharmacol* (1998) **53**:649–55.

39. Li Q, Wichems C, Heils A, Lesch KP, Murphy DL, Reduction in the density and expression, but not G-protein coupling, of serotonin receptors (5–HT1A) in 5-HT transporter knock-out mice: gender and brain region differences, *J Neurosci* (2000) **20**:7888–95.

40. Persico AM, Mengual E, Mössner R, et al, Barrel pattern formation requires serotonin uptake by thalamocortical endings, and not vesicular monoamine release, *J Neurosci* (2001) **21**:6862–73.

41. Salichon N, Gaspar P, Upton AL, et al, Excessive activation of serotonin (5-HT) 1B receptors disrupts the formation of sensory maps in monoamine oxidase A and 5-HT transporter knock-out mice, *J Neurosci* (2001) **21**:884–96.

42. Ramos A, Mormede P, Stress and emotionality: a multidimensional and genetic approach, *Neurosci Biobehav Rev* (1998) **22**:33–57.

43. Kendler KS, Walters EE, Neale MC, Kessler RC, Heath AC, Eaves LJ, The structure of the genetic and environmental risk factors for six major psychiatric disorders in women. Phobia, generalized anxiety disorder, panic disorder, bulimia, major depression, and alcoholism, *Arch Gen Psychiatry* (1995) **52**:374–83.

44. Higley JD, Suomi SJ, Linnoila M, CSF monoamine metabolite concentrations vary according to age, rearing, and sex, and are influenced by the stressor of social separation in rhesus monkeys, *Psychopharmacology* (1991) **103**:551–6.

45. Higley JD, Suomi SJ, Linnoila M, A longitudinal assessment of CSF monoamine metabolite and plasma cortisol concentrations in young rhesus monkeys, *Biol Psychiatry* (1992) **32**:127–45.

46. Bennett AJ, Lesch KP, Heils A, et al, Early experience and serotonin transporter gene variation interact to influence primate CNS function, *Mol Psychiatry* (2002) 7:118–22.

47. Kagan J, Reznick JS, Snidman N, Biological bases of childhood shyness, *Science* (1988) **240**:167–71.

48. Kagan J, Temperamental contributions to social behavior, *Am Psychol* (1989) 44:664–8.

49. Champoux M, Bennett A, Lesch KP, et al, Serotonin transporter gene polymorphism and neurobehavioral development in rhesus monkey neonates, *Soc Neurosci Abstr* (1999) **25**:69.

50. Champoux M, Bennett A, Shannon C, et al, Serotonin transporter gene polymorphism and behavior in rhesus monkey neonates, *Mol Psychiatry*, in press.

51. McPherson JD et al, A physical map of the human genome, *Nature* (2001) **409**:934–41.

52. Sachidanandam R, Weissman D, Schmidt SC, et al, A map of human genome sequence variation containing 1.42 million single nucleotide polymorphisms, *Nature* (2001) **409**:928–33.

53. Bacanu SA, Devlin B, Roeder K, The power of genomic control, *Am J Human Genet* (2000) **66**:1933–44.

54. Pritchard JK, Stephens M, Rosenberg NA, Donnelly P, Association mapping in structured populations, *Am J Human Genet* (2000) **67**:170–81.

55. Charney DS, Deutch A, A functional neuroanatomy of anxiety and fear: implications for the pathophysiology and treatment of anxiety disorders, *Crit Rev Neurobiol* (1996) **10**:419–46.

7

Generalized Anxiety Disorder Across Cultures

Dan J Stein and Hisato Matsunaga

Introduction

There is growing evidence that generalized anxiety disorder (GAD) is an independent disorder, prevalent across a range of countries,[1] and accompanied by substantial suffering and impairment. At the same time, there have been significant advances in understanding the psychobiology of anxiety disorders in general, and of GAD in particular. Pharmacotherapy and psychotherapy theoretically reverse the specific psychobiological dysfunctions that characterize GAD, and are certainly effective in its management.

There has not, however, been as much progress made in attempting to delineate psychosocial factors and cross-cultural issues that are germane to GAD. Advances in individual pharmacotherapy and psychotherapy have overshadowed work showing that GAD involves particular psychosocial risk factors. Further, the facts that GAD was first delineated by a Western nosology and that the bulk of studies have been undertaken in relatively few countries raise questions about the universality of this condition; at first blush it might be suggested that this is a 'culture-bound' disorder, restricted to only certain industrialized countries.

This chapter will focus on these kinds of psychosocial and cross-cultural issues. We begin by outlining three different theoretical approaches to cross-cultural psychiatry.[2,3] These approaches are not intended to subsume the work of any particular author, rather we hope that they have some heuristic value in allowing a conceptual framework for considering a range of relevant data. Indeed, once we have outlined the contrasting approaches, we use this framework to consider a number of current findings on generalized anxiety disorder.

Clinical position

A clinical position is based on a positivist approach to science.[4] In this view knowledge involves understanding the facts of the world, and science attempts to uncover the invariant relationships, or laws, between the phenomena of the world. Similarly, in psychological science, data are theory-neutral and explanations take the form of theorems which involve deductive-nomological systems.

In the medical arena, this position focuses on the phenomena of 'disease'. Biomedical knowledge involves the development of operational definitions in order to classify facts of the world, and the uncovering of contingent relationships between events.[5] From this perspective, scientific concepts of disease are value-free.[6]

In psychiatry, a clinical position readily applies Western nosologies to diverse populations. Kraepelin, for example, noted that the form of schizophrenia was similar in German patients and in Java. Thus psychotic symptomatology had universal forms which were biologically determined, but diverse contents which were colored by cultural factors.

The strength of the clinical approach lies in its attempt to extend a particular theoretical framework to diverse settings. The position highlights the scientific process of nosology construction. Arguably international employment of the American Psychiatric Association's Diagnostic and Statistical Manual (DSM) system by researchers who have adopted this position, for example, has allowed the work of different clinicians to converge, and has contributed to increased knowledge of psychiatric disorders.

Nevertheless, this position may be criticized on a number of fronts. Routine application of one theoretical framework may prevent the nosologist from recognizing the existence, or appreciating the character, of unfamiliar categories and symptoms. Conversely, this approach downplays the possible contribution that cross-cultural theories and methods make in helping us recognize the particular sociocultural influences on our own nosology.

Anthropological position

In contrast, an anthropological position draws on a hermeneutic approach to science. A hermeneutic approach emphasizes that science itself is a social practice, and that any scientific theory is ultimately only one form of subjective understanding. Psychological science is concerned not simply with explaining human behavior, but rather with understanding its meaning. Data are theory-laden and explanations involve interpretive understanding.

In the medical arena, this position focuses on 'illness', or the subjective perception and experience of a disease. Patients' explanatory models of disease are crucially influenced by their culture, and in turn inform the expression and experience of disease conditions. Analogously, professionals' explanatory models are ultimately cultural artifacts, and are value-laden.

In psychiatry, an anthropological position emphasizes the significant differences in patients from time to time and place and place, and the way in which distress is articulated within particular cultural idioms. The psychiatric anthropologist will note the existence, for example, of 'culture-bound' conditions that are limited to a particular time and place.

The strength of the anthropological approach lies in its emphasis on the relationship between psychiatric nosology and the social forms in which it is produced. It points to the importance of considering the ways in which cultural factors determine the experience and perception of mental disorder (rather than simply influencing its form). Clinical anthropologists have arguably made an important contribution by bringing this self-reflexive position to the practice of medicine.[7]

However, the anthropological position may have a number of significant flaws. A view of mental illness as merely social construction undermines the existence of psychiatric disorders as real phenomena which are generated by biopsychosocial mechanisms. Similarly, a view of nosology as simply a cultural product undermines the importance of scientific explanation as a valid process both in psychiatric research and clinical work.

Synthetic position

A synthetic or 'clinical anthropological' position attempts to combine the best of the clinical and anthropological positions. Although science is necessarily a social practice, it is also an attempt to explain the phenomena of the world by discovering the causal mechanisms that generate such phenomena.[8] Although data are theory-laden, in both natural and social sciences scientific progress occurs as the entities and mechanisms of the world are delineated.

In applying a synthetic position to medicine, it is important to focus on both disease and illness. We need to understand both the biological and psychosocial mechanisms that underpin medical conditions. In working with individual patients, we need to understand the objective aspects of their disorders, as well as peoples' subjective understanding and experience.

In psychiatry, a synthetic position similarly attempts to encompass both the subjective and objective aspects of suffering from a mental disorder. While classifications such as the DSM are necessarily sociocultural products, they allow a knowledge of real entities. As we increase our knowledge of the biological and psychosocial mechanisms that produce psychiatric disorders, so this knowledge becomes incorporated into psychiatric nosology.

The strength of this approach is that it has a place for both scientific knowledge and meaning construction. The reality of disease

and its biopsychosocial underpinnings is emphasized, while the expression and experience of illness within a particular sociocultural context is also incorporated. Such a view may be advantageous in thinking through various issues in cross-cultural psychiatry and cross-cultural aspects of the anxiety disorders.[2,3,9,10]

It is possible that many have implicitly adopted this 'clinical anthropological' position. Clinicians who use Western psychiatric categories in non-Western settings often acknowledge the limitations of these categories. Anthropologists who explore illness meanings in non-Western settings often acknowledge the scientific validity of biomedical knowledge of diseases. The DSM system is clearly a product of our own society, but advances in knowledge of real entities and processes will strengthen future editions.

GAD as disease

Can GAD be conceptualized as a biomedical disorder, that is found across cultures, and that is mediated by specific psychobiological processes? Certainly, the assumption of the DSM system is that this is indeed the case. On the other hand, the introduction of GAD into this official nosology was only relatively recent, and the disorder was initially seen as a residual diagnosis, to be made only once other conditions had been excluded.

There have been relatively few cross-cultural studies of GAD. A primary care study found that there were considerable differences across 14 countries, with 1-month prevalence of tenth edition International Classification of Diseases (ICD-10) GAD ranging from 1.0% (in Turkey) to 22.6% (in Brazil).[11] Nevertheless, the validity of the GAD construct was demonstrated by a strong and consistent association between tension and worry on the one hand, and related somatic symptoms on the other.

Furthermore, a more recent synthesis of data from community studies in several countries found that DSM-III-R (3rd, revised edition) GAD had a similar prevalence, similar demographic features, and similar comorbidities and course.[1] DSM definitions may exclude a substantial proportion of people with clinically significant chronic anxiety,[12] and revising the duration requirement to 1 month may yield better discrimination between cases and non-cases in terms of impaired functioning.[11]

In community studies, GAD appears more common in unmarried than married people, and in low socioeconomic status (SES) than middle or high SES respondents.[13,14] However, sociodemographic variables (gender, race-ethnicity, marital status, SES status) are not significant predictors of the course of GAD in either epidemiological[12] or community[15] studies. Thus, marital status and socioeconomic achievement would appear to be influenced by GAD or its determinants rather than the other way around.

From a disease perspective, the range of symptoms in GAD is perhaps uncomfortably broad. Even if we accept that GAD is an independent disorder, it seems to be a particularly heterogeneous condition for which it is difficult to specify a unique 'behavioral marker'. One possibility is that GAD primarily involves 'tension'; a tension that is both psychological (anxious expectation) and somatic (muscle tension). Certainly, there is a growing understanding of the psychobiology of GAD (Nutt, this volume). GAD appears to be characterized by specific risk factors and by particular neuroanatomic and neurochemical abnormalities, which may underpin such psychological and somatic 'tension'. However, there is also significant overlap with findings from studies of depression and other anxiety

disorders. Thus, additional work needs to be done in order to delineate the specificity of psychobiological dysfunction in GAD.

GAD as illness

Might it be argued that GAD is primarily a social construction that reflects the particular context of the DSM system rather than any medical reality? Even if we accept the diagnosis of GAD as valid in the West, does diagnosis of GAD in non-Western countries entail a 'category fallacy' (analogous to diagnosing an Eastern condition, such as 'semen loss', in the West), which reifies Western classification as based on universal natural kinds.

Certainly, as noted earlier, in DSM-III, GAD was seen as a residual diagnosis to be made only when better-delineated conditions such as panic disorder and depression had been excluded. Furthermore, there has been considerable flux in the diagnostic criteria for GAD over the years. On the other hand, there is growing evidence in support of the argument that GAD is, at least in the West, an independent and disabling disorder.

One interesting aspect of community and clinical data on GAD is the relatively consistent finding that the disorder is much more common in women.[12,16] While it may be argued that this reflects the existence of particular psychobiological risk factors in females, another view might be that GAD is a relatively gender-specific way of expressing distress (with internalizing symptoms predominating over externalizing ones in women, and externalizing symptoms more common in men). Similar logic may apply to some racial-ethnic differences in the prevalence of GAD.[13,14,17,18]

It is also interesting to note that DSM revisions have seen a growing emphasis on 'worry' in relation to GAD. This would arguably seem to be a particularly Western kind of focus; in many other cultures anxiety symptoms are expressed in predominantly somatic rather than psychological terms. Even in Western primary care settings, 'somatizers' (who more commonly have GAD than depression) are more common than 'psychologizers' (who more commonly have depression than GAD).[19]

To date there have been relatively few cross-cultural studies of worry.[20] Interestingly, some of the work that has been done suggests that worry per se is not necessarily related to poor health – a cross-national study suggested that worries about the self and close others (micro worries) were related to poor health, whereas worries about society or the entire world (macro worries) were not.[21]

Furthermore, the DSM concept of 'excessive worry' may be particularly difficult to determine in many non-Western contexts, where lack of finances and resources may be more likely to be real concerns. Hispanic patients with GAD could not be differentiated clinically, for example, from those with anxiety not otherwise specified (who do not meet criteria for 'excessive worry').[22]

In addition, in epidemiological studies across countries, the association between GAD and low SES is stronger with ICD criteria (which do not require that worry is excessive or unrealistic) than DSM criteria (where the inclusion of this criterion seems unnecessarily restrictive for those people, such as people of low SES, who do in fact face difficult life circumstances).[12]

Is there evidence that the expression and experience of anxiety vary from place to place? A range of research supports this idea.[23,24,25,26,27] For example, there are reports from different parts of the world of a range of different conditions in which anxiety symptoms predominate, but in somewhat different ways, including ataque in Hispanics,[28] brain fag in Nigeria,[29] neurasthenia in China,[7] and shinkeishitsu in Japan.[30]

Similarly, certain Japanese authors have suggested that GAD in Japan may be characterized by symptoms not emphasized in DSM-IV; these include loss of volition and avoidance of emotional experience. Indeed, a study of Japanese psychology students found that they had significant difficulty in reliably identifying GAD, but not other anxiety and mood disorders,[31] which the authors felt to be consistent with cross-cultural variations in the experience of anxiety. Research exploring differences in help-seeking behavior across cultures in patients with chronic anxiety would contribute usefully to this discussion.

A synthetic view of GAD

Is it possible to synthesize some of the contrasting considerations that support a view of GAD as either a 'disease' or an 'illness'? Despite the relative lack of cross-cultural data on GAD, a reading of the literature perhaps allows an integrative approach which posits the presence of specific psychobiological features which characterize anxiety symptoms across cultures, but which also puts forward a view of symptomatology that is sufficiently broad to encompass the experience of a wide range of patients.

GAD can arguably be characterized as a tension disorder, with patients experiencing both psychological and somatic tension. Freud's early description of 'anxiety neurosis' patients, with free-floating anxiety accompanied by somatic symptoms, retains its relevance. More recent work has emphasized that muscle tension in particular is important in differentiating GAD from other anxiety disorders and from depression.[32]

Although GAD may be seen independently of major depressive disorder, community studies demonstrate how commonly GAD is temporally followed by the latter disorder.[12] Indeed, the triad of anxiety-somatization-depression may be posited to be a universal psychiatric phenomenon, highly prevalent in a broad range of different historical periods and contemporary cultures. This is particularly apparent in primary care settings.[33] Importantly, comorbidity of GAD with depression is particularly disabling.

GAD may be characterized not only by specific neurobiological factors (Nutt, this volume), but also by particular psychosocial ones, such as stressful events.[34] Arguably, life events may simply be perceived as more stressful in GAD.[35] Nevertheless, twin data show that environmental risk factors differ considerably in GAD and in major depression,[36] consistent with findings that certain life events predispose to anxiety while others predispose to depression.[37,38]

There are several possible explanations (ranging from neurobiological to psychosocial) of why anxiety is so commonly followed by depression.[39,40] However, given the sometimes lengthy course of this progression, proving particular hypotheses is challenging. Perhaps we can look forward to further progress in delineating the specific psychobiology of GAD and anxiety-somatization-depression in future years.

As discussed in the previous section, the experience and expression of anxiety and of tension may, however, vary from time to time and place to place. Thus, for example, different cultures may preferentially choose different somatic pathways as the predominant idioms of distress. Clinicians need to be aware of such differences in order to optimize appropriate diagnosis, to facilitate the doctor–patient relationship, and to enhance adherence to inverventions.

Psychologizing symptoms may be particularly common in patients in the West, both in GAD (e.g. 'worry') and in depression (e.g. 'ruminations'). Another possibility, however, is that worry is not a primary feature of GAD, but is rather merely one kind of secondary avoidance behavior (Borkovec, this volume); a number of factors operating in the West may make this form of avoidance more common in this context. More empirical work is needed to differentiate between, and substantiate, these hypotheses.

Conclusion

Aspects of DSM-IV GAD (such as the focus on worry) may be particularly relevant to Western contexts. Nevertheless, a condition characterized by psychological and somatic tension is prevalent in a range of cultures,[1,11] and the diagnosis of GAD in non-Western cultures cannot easily be termed a 'category fallacy'. Furthermore, the triad of anxiety-somatization-depression is arguably a universally important psychiatric phenomenon, and is particularly important in primary care settings.[33]

The psychobiological underpinnings of GAD and of anxiety-somatization-depression are gradually being defined. Evolutionary considerations might suggest the usefulness of a system that is activated under conditions of stress, and which ensures close attention to future possibilities as well as somatic hyperarousal.[41] Advances in cognitive and affective neuroscience aim to allow the proximal mechanisms that activate this putative alarm system to be better delineated in the future.

Cross-cultural approaches to GAD have an important role in both clinical and research arenas. In our multi-cultural world, clinicians need to be aware of differences in the expression of anxiety in order to optimize diagnosis and management of patients from a wide range of backgrounds. In addition, cross-cultural theories and methods may ultimately help lead to improvements in the diagnostic criteria for GAD and in the symptom measures used to assess its severity.

Acknowledgement

Dr Stein is supported by the Medical Research Council of South Africa.

References

1. Kessler RC, Andrade L, Bijl RV et al., The effects of comorbidity on the onset and persistence of generalized anxiety disorder in the ICPE surveys, *Psychological Medicine* (in press)
2. Stein DJ, Cross-cultural psychiatry and the DSM-IV, *Compr Psychiatry* (1993) 34:322–9
3. Stein DJ, Matsunaga H, Cross-cultural aspects of social anxiety disorder, *Psychiatr Clin North Am* (2001) 24:773–82
4. Stein DJ, Philosophy and the DSM-III, *Compr Psychiatry* (1991) 32:404–15
5. Hempel CG, *Aspects of Scientific Explanation and Other Essays in the Philosophy of Science* (New York: Free Press, 1965)
6. Boorse C, On the distinction between disease and illness, *Philosophy and Public Affairs* (2001) 5:49–68
7. Kleinman A, *Rethinking Psychiatry: From Cultural Category to Personal Experience* (New York: Free Press, 1988)
8. Bhaskar R, *A Realist Theory of Science*, 2nd edn. (Sussex: Harvester Press, 1978)
9. Stein DJ, Rapoport JL, Cross-cultural studies and obsessive-compulsive disorder, *CNS Spectrums* (1996) 1:42–6
10. Stein DJ, Williams D, Cross-cultural aspects of anxiety disorders. In: Stein DJ, Hollander E, *Textbook of Anxiety Disorders* (Washington, DC: American Psychiatric Press, 2001)
11. Maier W, Gansicke A, Freyberger HJ et al., Generalized anxiety disorder (ICD-10) in primary care from a cross-cultural perspective: a valid diagnostic entity? *Acta Psychiatr Scand* (2000) 101:29–36
12. Kessler RC, The epidemiology of pure and comorbid generalized anxiety disorder. A review and evaluation of recent research, *Acta Psychiatr Scand* (2001) 406(Suppl) 7–13
13. Blazer DG, Hughes D, George L et al., Generalized anxiety disorder. In: Robins LN, Regier DA, *Psychiatric Disorders in America* (New York: The Free Press, 1991) 180–203
14. Wittchen H-U, Zhao S, Kessler RC et al., DSM-III-R generalized anxiety disorder in the National Comorbidity Survey, *Arch Gen Psychiatry* (1994) 51:355–64
15. Yonkers KA, Dyck IR, Warshaw MKMB, Factors predicting the clinical course of generalised anxiety disorder, *Br J Psychiatry* (2000) 176:544–9
16. Howell HB, Brawman-Mintzer O, Monnier J et al., Generalized anxiety disorder in women, *Psych Clin North Am* (2001) 24:165–78
17. Karno M, Golding JM, Burnam MA et al., Anxiety disorders among Mexican Americans and non-Hispanic whites in Los Angeles, *J Nerv Ment Dis* (1989) 177:202–9
18. Mavreas VG, Bebbington PE, Greeks, British Greek Cypriots and Londoners: A comparison of morbidity, *Psychol Med* (1988) 18:433–42
19. Bridget K, Goldberg D, Evans B et al., Determinants of somatization in primary care, *Psychol Med* (1991) 21:473–83
20. Watari KF, Brodbeck C, Culture, health, and financial appraisals: Comparison of worry in older Japanese Americans and European Americans, *J Clin Geropsychology* (2000) 6:25–9
21. Boehnke K, Schwartz S, Stromberg C et al., The structure and dynamics of worry: theory, measurement, and cross-national replications, *J Pers* (1998) 66:745–82
22. Street LL, Salman E, Garfinkle R et al., Differentiating between generalized anxiety disorder and anxiety disorder not otherwise specified in a Hispanic population: is it only a matter of worry? *Depress Anxiety* (1997) 5:1–6
23. Friedman S, *Cultural Issues in the Treatment of Anxiety* (New York, NY: Guilford Press, 1997)
24. Good BJ, Kleinman AM, Culture and anxiety: Cross-cultural evidence for the patterning of anxiety disorders. In: Tuma AH, Maser JD, *Anxiety and the Anxiety Disorders* (Hillsdale, NJ: Erlbaum, 1985)

25. Guarnaccia PJ, Kirmayer LJ, Culture and the anxiety disorders. In: Widiger TA, Frances A, Pincus HA, First MB, Davis W, *DSM-IV Sourcebook, Vol 3.* (Washington, DC: American Psychiatric Press, 1997)

26. Neal AM, Turner SM, Anxiety disorders research with African Americans: Current status, *Psychol Bull* (1991) **109**:400–10

27. Spielberger C, Diaz-Guerrero R, *Cross Cultural Anxiety* (London: Taylor & Francis, 1990)

28. Liebowitz MR, Salman E, Jusino CM et al., Ataque de nervios and panic disorder. *Am J Psychiatry* (1994) **151**:871–5

29. Simons RC, Hughes CC, *The Culture-Bound Syndromes* (Dordrecht: Reidel, 1985)

30. Kitanishi K, Mori A, Morita therapy: 1919 to 1995, *Psychiatry Clin Neurosci* (1995) **49**:245–54

31. Sugiura T, Hasui C, Aoki Y et al., Japanese psychology students as psychiatric diagnosticians: Application of criteria of mood and anxiety disorders to written case vignettes using the RDC and DSM-IV, *Psychol Rep* (1998) **82**:771–81

32. Joormann J, Stöber J, Somatic symptoms of generalized anxiety disorder for the DSM-IV: Associations with pathological worry and depression symptoms in a nonclinical sample, *J Anxiety Disord* (1999) **13**:491–503

33. Gureje O, Simon GE, Ustun TB et al., Somatization in cross-cultural perspective: A World Health Organization study in primary care, *Am J Psychiatry* (1997) **154**:989–95

34. Blazer D, Hughes D, George LK, Stressful life events and the onset of a generalized anxiety syndrome, *Am J Psychiatry* (1987) **144**:1178–83

35. Brantley PJ, Mehan DJJ, Ames SC et al., Minor stressors and generalized anxiety disorder among low-income patients attending primary care clinics, *J Nerv Ment Dis* (1999) **187**:435–40

36. Kendler KS, Neale MC, Kessler RC et al., Major depression and generalized anxiety disorder: Same genes, (partly) different environments? *Arch Gen Psychiatry* (1992) **49**:716–22

37. Finlay-Jones R, Brown GW, Types of stressful life events and the onset of anxiety and depressive disorders, *Psychol Med* (1981) **11**:803–15

38. Monroe SM, Psychosocial factors in anxiety and depression. In: Maser JD, Cloninger CR, *Comorbidity of Mood and Anxiety Disorders* (Washington, DC: American Psychiatric Press Inc, 1990) 463–97

39. Akiskal HS, Anxiety: Definition, relationship to depression, and proposal for an integrative model. In: Tuma AH, Maser JD, *Anxiety and the Anxiety Disorders.* (Hillsdale, NJ: Lawrence Earlbaum Associates, 1985) 787–97

40. Stein DJ, Hollander E, *Textbook of Anxiety Disorders* (Washington, DC: American Psychiatric Press, 2001)

41. Stein DJ, Bouwer C, A neuro-evolutionary approach to the anxiety disorders, *J Anxiety Disord* (1997) **11**:409–29

III   Treatment

8

Psychological Aspects and Treatment of Generalized Anxiety Disorder

Thomas D Borkovec

Characteristics of worry and GAD

Worry involves thinking

Worry, a central and defining psychological process in generalized anxiety disorder (GAD), primarily involves verbal-linguistic (as opposed to imaginal) cognitive activity. People are mainly talking to themselves when they are worrying and are less likely to engage in imagery. This has been demonstrated for GAD clients (often at rest as well as during worry episodes) in thought-sampling reports,[1] in assessments of verbal and spatial working memory,[2] and in elevated left frontal cortical activity.[3] In treated GAD clients, both their ratio of reported thoughts and images[4] and their cortical functioning[3] have been found to move toward normalization after successful psychotherapy. Moreover, healthy normals frequently show the same types of evidence of increased thought and decreased imagery when they worry in a laboratory setting. The content and associated mental processes of worry have also been shown to reflect a high degree of abstraction compared to the more concrete and imagery-eliciting contents of the mental activity associated with thinking about nonworrisome topics,[5] and the degree of concreteness of the worry content also normalizes (increases) after psychotherapy.[6] The distinction between thought and imagery is a functionally important one: emotional content represented in imagery elicits significant sympathetic autonomic nervous system activity, whereas the same content represented mentally in words has little autonomic effect.[7] Imagery is closely tied to efferent command in physiological response and affect; thought is not. Thus, these different cognitive ways of dealing with emotionally balanced material are likely to have very different implications for the processing of emotion, as we will see below, and potentially for understanding the development, maintenance, and treatment of GAD.

Worry begets more worry

Worry incubates. That is, it leads to a strengthening of the tendency to worry and there is an increase in subsequent negative thought intrusions after one has engaged in a brief period of worry.[8] This effect occurs in both chronic worriers and nonworriers, and it occurs despite the fact that no environmental events have transpired during the worrying that might cause a strengthening of anxious meanings or facilitate the development of intrusive thoughts. It also appears that worrying itself can contribute to a spreading of anxious meanings to previously neutral stimuli. When threatening words (inherent to the content of worrisome thinking) are repeatedly paired with a neutral stimulus, GAD clients alone and not nonanxious controls display a defensive cardiovascular response to each threat word presentation, and over time only the GAD clients develop an orienting response to the neutral stimulus.[9] Such conditioning processes may well underlie the further development of the hypervigilance so characteristic of GAD.

Worry is believed to have benefits

GAD clients believe that worry does serve beneficial purposes.[10] They feel that it can prevent bad events from happening (both actually and superstitiously), that it prepares them for the worst, and that it motivates them and facilitates problem-solving. Nonanxious people believe that worry can serve these same purposes to the same extent. GAD clients are, however, distinguished from healthy normals by their significantly greater belief that worrying distracts them from more emotional topics, topics about which they do not want to think.

GAD is characterized by selective information processing

A considerable amount of research applying the experimental methods of cognitive psychology has now demonstrated that GAD is associated with specific types of biases in information processing (see MacLeod[11] for an excellent and comprehensive review of this literature).

Attentional bias

Clients with GAD show an attentional bias, even without conscious awareness, to a wide variety of threatening information.[12] Similar investigations of other anxiety disorders[13,14] have not routinely shown such a bias, and when threat bias has been seen, it has usually been associated with disorder-specific stimuli rather than a broad range of threatening material.[15] Interestingly, research participants not diagnosed with GAD but scoring high on measures of trait anxiety tend to display attentional bias to threat only when stressed.[16] Based on the findings from these various investigations of selective attention, MacLeod[11] speculates that the preferential allocation of attentional resources to threat during the encoding of environmental information may play a significant role in the development of chronic anxiety in vulnerable individuals and in the maintenance of anxiety in those already suffering from GAD.

Interpretive bias

GAD clients also display an interpretive bias when the information presented is ambiguous with regard to its threatening or nonthreatening meaning.[17] Thus, if a stimulus can be interpreted either as representing a danger or as reflecting something benign, individuals with GAD are likely to choose or generate a more threatening meaning than nonanxious people. Like the attentional bias results, people with other anxiety disorders show this type of interpretive bias mainly when the information is relevant and specific to their disorder,[18] whereas GAD clients see such dangers in a wide variety of situations.

Explicit and implicit memory retrieval

Although GAD clients can show a tendency to report more negative information when asked to recall past autobiographical events,[19] they do not usually recall[20] or recognize[21] threatening information presented briefly during laboratory tasks to any greater degree than nonanxious people. They have, however, been found to recall previously presented threat words more than nonanxious people if the duration of exposure to the words is long (8 seconds).[22] Although people with social phobias[20] and specific phobias[23] have failed to display any retrieval bias, those with panic disorder, obsessive-compulsive disorder, and post-traumatic stress disorder have shown this type of bias.[20,24,25]

Some evidence suggests that GAD may be specifically associated with a greater implicit memory bias for threat,[26] whereas the other anxiety disorders are not so characterized.[27] Because this GAD effect has not always been replicated, MacLeod[11] concludes that one must be less confident in the possibility of an implicit memory retrieval bias in GAD than in its clear association with attentional and interpretive biases.

Effects of therapy and training on selective processing

Finally, evidence exists to suggest that the information biases present in GAD can play a causal role in the development of anxiety. For example, successful cognitive-behavioral treatments targeting cognitive activity result in reductions in the selective processing of threat.[28] Indeed, the degree to which such a reduction occurs correlates with the degree of clinical improvement. This is in contrast to the effects of benzodiazepine therapy which reduces anxiety symptoms but has no effect on the processing of threatening information.[29] Moreover, recent efforts to experimentally train cognitive biases[30] have demonstrated not only that biases can be taught but that the creation of a bias toward threat leads to increases in state anxiety and/or anxiety vulnerability to the occurrence of subsequent stressors.

Worry and GAD are characterized by muscle tension and reduced autonomic variability

GAD clients are also characterized by an interesting psychophysiology. Even at rest, they display greater muscle tension and reduced autonomic variability compared to nonanxious people, and engaging in challenging tasks or in worry results in further phasic reductions in cardiovascular variability and parasympathetic tone.[31,32] Even nonanxious people show these effects when they worry. Such a psychophysiology is the likely explanation for the empirical findings that led to the DSM-IV decision to reduce the earlier DSM-III-R associated symptoms for GAD from 18 to the current 6. These 6 symptoms (restlessness/keyed up/on edge, difficulty concentrating, muscle tension, insomnia, fatigability, and irritability) were found to be the most frequently and reliably reported somatic experiences among GAD clients.[33] Interestingly, each of these symptoms is to a greater degree a reflection of central nervous system activity than are the 11 autonomically mediated symptoms deleted from the GAD associated symptom checklist. Although several of these 6 symptoms overlap with symptom criteria for mood disorders, muscle tension has been shown to be particularly distinctive of GAD when compared to other anxiety and mood disorders.[34]

Why variability in autonomic activity might be reduced, both in the tonic state of GAD and in the phasic state of a worrisome episode, is reasonably explained by the conditions that GAD clients face. Unlike all of the other anxiety disorders much of the time, there is no effective motoric avoidance response that can be made to eliminate a perceived threat. Worry is about nonexistent, future, possible threats, threats that have been shown empirically to have a very low probability of actually happening anyway.[35] When perception of threat occurs, sympathetic fight-or-flight is a natural response. In the case of phobias, panic disorder, or obsessive-compulsive disorder, behavioral avoidance of external situations related to the fear readily develops and is negatively reinforced by successful, temporary removal of both the feared situation and the distressing anxiety symptoms triggered by the situation. In the case of GAD, however, there is nowhere to flee and no one to fight. Neither sympathetic activation nor autonomic variability (a generally adaptive parasympathetically mediated characteristic[32]) are needed to facilitate flight or fight and are thus apparently suppressed. It is interesting to note that several experimental laboratory tasks (mental arithmetic, recall of a past aversive event, threat of shock, and isometric grip tasks) which cause phasic reductions in parasympathetic tone in healthy normals closely reflect several of the common characteristics of the GAD client.[36] Given these circumstances, the better evolutionarily based model for GAD may well be found in the 'freezing' response, so typical of animals confronting danger without the opportunity to escape. This response may relate to the frequent procrastinations commonly reported by GAD clients as well as the lengthened decision-making latencies of chronic worriers when reaction times to simple visual discriminations are assessed in the laboratory.[37] Finally, the discovery of lowered vagal tone in GAD will likely be significant in our eventual understanding of the attentional bias effects described earlier for this disorder, given that vagal tone has been implicated in adaptive attentional control.[38]

Reduced parasympathetic tone is not unique to GAD; the same phenomenon has been found in some of the other anxiety disorders (e.g., in panic disorder[39]). On the other hand, it may be the case that the reduced autonomic variability sometimes observed in other anxiety disorders is the specific effect of the apprehensive expectation (i.e., worry) that is pervasive across all of the anxiety disorders, even though it is the central feature of GAD.

Behavioral aspects of GAD

While the other anxiety disorders tend to be characterized by specific, circumscribed feared situations, GAD clients usually respond with anxiety and worry to a very broad array of stimuli, as demonstrated in the information-processing research described earlier and in the fact that GAD is associated with significantly greater amounts of worry over miscellaneous topics.[40] Partly as a consequence of this and partly as a consequence of living in a world where nonexistent potential dangers cannot be physically avoided, behavioral avoidance is not such an obvious feature of GAD as it is of other anxiety disorders. As mentioned earlier, however, decision-making latencies are slowed in GAD. Indeed, induced states of worry cause such retardation even in nonanxious individuals.[37] Furthermore, subtle avoidance behaviors can be detected if clients are carefully interviewed,[41] and GAD clients have been found to engage in a variety of behaviors designed to prevent catastrophes from happening.[42]

Avoidant functions of worry and the maintenance of GAD

Given that the threats for GAD clients largely exist only in the future and so cannot be behaviorally avoided, it makes sense that people with GAD would use their cognitive capabilities to try to prevent catastrophes from happening. Indeed, the thought system likely evolved to anticipate the future and to engage in problem-solving in order to minimize bad events and maximize good events.[43] The information-processing literature reviewed above indicates that GAD clients perceive a considerable amount of danger in their future environments, and so they are understandably motivated to worry in an attempt to figure out how to avoid catastrophe and/or prepare for the worst.

Considerable evidence suggests that worry does indeed function as a cognitive avoidance response to threatening information.[44] Like any avoidance response, worry prevents emotional processing of the affective material that could otherwise lead to anxiety reduction; indeed, its occurrence maintains or further strengthens the anxiety. For example, worry by individuals with phobia for public speaking just prior to the repeated presentation of a phobic image eliminates cardiovascular responses to that image, in contrast to the large cardiovascular responses to images presented just after relaxed thinking. Such findings indicate that worry is likely negatively reinforced by the phasic reduction or removal of aversive (somatically anxious) states it produces in the presence of threatening material. Worrying just before actual, repeated presentations of a threatening event (public speaking) also leads to maintained subjective anxiety, in contrast to gradually declining levels of anxiety over repeated exposures among speech phobics who engage in relaxing thinking. Worrying just after viewing a stressful film results in significantly greater amounts of cogni-

tive intrusion during subsequent days than does relaxing or imagining the content of the film just after seeing it. Finally, as mentioned earlier, GAD clients report a belief that their worrying functions to avoid catastrophes. They believe that it can actually prevent such events (either superstitiously or by effective problem-solving) or that it can minimize the emotional impact of any bad events that do occur. Each of these beliefs creates conditions sufficient for the occurrence of negative reinforcement of the worrying itself. For example, given that very few bad events about which people worry actually occur, the worrying of a GAD client is most commonly followed by the nonoccurrence of the feared event, and the tendency to worry is thus strengthened because of its frequent association with the perceived prevention of bad events (see also Chapter 4).

Psychotherapy for worry and GAD

We have learned a considerable amount about the nature and functions of worry and GAD. The psychotherapies that have been created to treat GAD have been based on such knowledge, and promising new developments stemming from recent empirical observations are being explored. The next section will describe the most commonly used techniques, summarize the extant outcome literature evaluating their efficacy, and discuss new approaches to GAD treatment that are in the initial stage of development.

Customary cognitive behavioral therapy for GAD

The most common psychotherapy for worry and GAD involves the application of a combination of cognitive and behavioral therapy methods (CBT). Because GAD is not characterized by discrete environmental fear triggers and associated behavioral avoidance responses, the usual exposure methods found to be so effective with other anxiety disorders are not as central to its treatment. Instead, the primary goal of this therapy is to provide the client with cognitive and behavioral coping responses to practice and use whenever incipient anxiety is detected in daily life.

Cognitive therapy

Because GAD involves the pervasive perception of threat, frequent predictions of catastrophes, and self-strengthening worry, cognitive therapy has long been employed to help clients to shift from worrisome activity to perceiving the world, the future, and themselves in a more accurate manner. The therapist and client work together to identify how the client is perceiving events in an anxious way, to evaluate the accuracy of those perceptions through logic and evidence, and to create alternative perspectives that can be generated whenever the client detects worry, anxiety, and the cognitive interpretations that give rise to that perception of threat. Clients can also be encouraged to keep records of their worries, what they are predicting might occur, and what the actual outcome turns out to be in order to create a history of evidence concerning the accuracy of their predictions and of the alternative ways of predicting.

Behavior therapy

Because of their chronically elevated muscle tension and deficient parasympathetic tone, the most common behavioral intervention for GAD involves relaxation training and application. Clients are taught various methods for producing relaxation responses (e.g., progressive muscular relaxation; slowed, paced diaphragmatic breathing; relaxing imagery; and meditational techniques) and are encouraged to make use of these in daily life, both in response to incipient anxiety or worry and frequently throughout the day even when they are not anxious. This type of applied relaxation training (developed by Öst) aims at helping clients specifically to intervene and stop the spiralling of anxiety responses and generally to cultivate a more relaxed lifestyle. Systematic exposure to anxiety-provoking situations can be employed if such discrete situations can be identified, but the goal of such exposures has less to do with engineering anxiety extinction processes and more to do with creating frequent opportunities to practice the deployment of coping responses until they become more habitual and effective in eliminating anxious responding. Sometimes stimulus control methods have also been incorporated into the above basic behavioral interventions in order to reduce both the frequency of self-strengthening worry and its association with multiple environmental circumstances. In this technique, clients are asked to (a) establish a worry period to take place at the same time each day and in the same place, (b) monitor their daily worrying and learn to detect its initiation, (c) postpone any worrying during the day until their worry period and at other times focus their attention back to the task at hand or to what is immediately present in their environment, and (d) make use of the worry period to practice the cognitive skills that they have been learning in therapy to create alternative, realistic views of the worrisome situation for use whenever they detect that worry during the day. Finally, because mood disorders or at least moderate depression are often comorbid with GAD, some CBT methods have included behavioral activation strategies wherein clients are encouraged to increase the number of pleasant activities in which they engage during the day.

Imagery rehearsal methods

Several techniques have been developed that make use of imagery rehearsals of the cognitive and relaxation responses that the clients are learning in therapy. Because worry and other anxiety processes are habitual and automatic (having been practiced by clients sometimes for many years), it is important for clients to frequently practice the alternative coping responses. Having clients rehearse the new responses in the therapy session, using imagined scenes of typical internal and environmental cues that commonly elicit their anxiety and worry, can facilitate the acquisition and strengthening of their new cognitive and relaxation responses and can increase the likelihood that clients will remember to rapidly deploy these responses upon detection of anxiety cues in their daily lives.

Outcome research on CBT for GAD

CBT has been the principal psychotherapy method that has been systematically evaluated in carefully controlled clinical trials of GAD. Reviews of the GAD therapy outcome research[45-47] have been consistent in their conclusions: CBT is indeed an effective form of psychological intervention, but great need exists for even more effective therapies to be developed. The findings of the most recent review and meta-analysis of this literature are summarized below, followed by a discussion of clinical trials that were published after this review was conducted.

Borkovec and Ruscio[46] evaluated the outcomes of 13 extant controlled trials of psychotherapy for GAD, both by examining the significant results within each study and by calculating effect sizes for conditions from 11 of these studies which provided sufficient statistical information to allow for effect size calculations. The majority of these 13 investigations, all of which included some form of CBT, were characterized by strong methodological features, including DSM diagnoses by semi-structured interviews, assessment of diagnostic reliability, 'blind' assessors, multiple therapists seeing clients in each of the compared therapy conditions, detailed protocol manuals with independent adherence checks, assessment of therapy credibility and expectancy for improvement to insure equivalence of conditions on these important nonspecific factors, and follow-up assessment averaging 9 months after the completion of therapy. Two-thirds of the clients were women, average age was 38.6 years, and average chronicity of GAD was 6.8 years. On average, 10.6 sessions of therapy were offered to clients, with a session averaging 69 minutes.

From examination of the results within each study, CBT was found to be significantly superior to (a) waiting-list no-treatment conditions in all 6 of such comparisons at post-therapy assessment, (b) conditions that controlled for nonspecific effects (placebo or alternative psychological interventions) in 9 of 11 comparisons at post-therapy and 7 of 9 comparisons at follow-up, and (c) conditions containing only the behavioral therapy or the cognitive therapy component alone in 2 of 10 post-therapy and 3 of 7 follow-up comparisons. These investigations also found that the clinical improvements experienced by the clients at post-therapy were generally maintained or increased at follow-up.

CBT showed the largest within-group effect sizes (post-therapy or follow-up mean minus pre-therapy mean divided by pre-therapy standard deviation) on both anxiety (mean = 2.46) and depression (mean = 1.18) measures compared to no-treatment (0.01 and 0.14), nonspecific conditions (2.05 and 0.92), and component conditions (1.72 and 0.95). Similarly, CBT yielded a large between-group effect size (CBT post-therapy or follow-up mean minus comparison condition mean divided by their pooled post-therapy standard deviation) when compared to no-treatment (1.09 for anxiety and 0.92 for depression, averaged over post-therapy and follow-up assessments) and moderate effect sizes when compared to nonspecific conditions (0.50 and 0.43, respectively) and component conditions (0.40 and 0.35, respectively). Attrition rates in these investigations have been relatively low (mean over studies = 14.8%), with CBT showing the lowest level (mean = 8.3%).

One final comment about the extant outcome literature is that there has not yet been an adequate trial contrasting psychological treatment with medication or evaluating their combination. Two investigations that did include diazepam treatments and found them to be inferior to CBT unfortunately used an ineffectual (fixed, low dose) regime for the medication.

Since the most recently published review of GAD therapy research, three additional controlled investigations have been conducted (one of which will be reviewed later). In one study,[48] cognitive therapy alone and behavior therapy alone were found to be equivalent in outcome, and their within-group effect sizes matched those of previously utilized component conditions. In a second study, outcome equivalence was demonstrated for cognitive therapy alone, applied relaxation and self-control desensitization, and a CBT combination of these techniques.[49] Interestingly, review of all component control investigations in this publication revealed that CBT has usually been found superior to one of its components in those studies using brief durations of treatment (mean = 9.2 hours), whereas equivalence is found when long-duration treatment (13.5 hours) is provided. It appears that sufficient learning of one set of psychological techniques

that target one domain of anxious responding (cognitive or somatic activity) can ultimately affect the other domain.

Despite the clear evidence supporting the specific efficacy of CBT in the treatment of GAD, this same literature also indicates that further treatment development is needed. Averaging over all investigations, one finds that only 50% of clients so treated meet high endstate criteria, i.e. are returned to within a standard deviation of nonanxious normative means on anxiety measures.[47] Learning to employ cognitive and somatic coping responses has been found to be insufficient for half of all treated GAD clients. Apparently, additional factors are involved in the maintenance of their disorder that have thus far not been adequately addressed by traditional CBT techniques. The final section of this chapter discusses new therapeutic directions designed to impact on other empirically demonstrated characteristics of GAD that may be causatively involved in the disorder.

New developments in the psychological treatment of GAD

One of the more recent outcome investigations reviewed above[49] also discovered that interpersonal problems remaining at the end of therapy negatively predicted post-therapy and follow-up improvement, suggesting that interpersonal processes may be implicated in the maintenance of GAD and that targeting such processes may be important in future therapy developments. Earlier research had anticipated this hypothesis. Worry has been empirically linked to social evaluative fears, social phobia is a common comorbid condition for GAD, interpersonal concerns are the most frequent worrisome topic, and GAD clients recall greater role-reversed relationships in childhood and cluster to a greater degree into three predominant interpersonal problem areas (dominant, vindictive, and overly nurturing) than do nonanxious people.[44] Moreover, one uncontrolled open trial of interpersonal psychotherapy for GAD offered promising results. All of the above findings have encouraged a controlled trial that is currently being conducted to compare CBT with and without the addition of an interpersonal therapy. This interpersonal component is designed to help clients to identify their interpersonal needs and to learn better ways of having those needs satisfied.[50] It is anticipated that successfully addressing interpersonal issues in therapy may add to the efficacy of the basic CBT intervention, and the hypothetical causal role of interpersonal problems in the etiology and/or maintenance of GAD would be supported if the combined treatment is indeed found to be superior to CBT alone.

Another recent direction involves the incorporation of mindfulness/acceptance training into the CBT approach.[51] The special features of this approach emphasize teaching clients to accept unwanted inner experience, engage in actions that represent personally valued directions of behavior regardless of inner experience, and focus on present moment experience as opposed to future-oriented worrisome thinking. This type of intervention has received preliminary empirical support from an uncontrolled open trial that included GAD clients[52] and from a small pilot investigation.[51]

Finally, based on recent research findings that GAD clients experience a greater degree of intolerance for uncertainty than people with other anxiety disorders,[53] along with poor problem-solving orientation,[54] inaccurate beliefs about the functions and effects of worry,[55] and lack of emotional processing of anxiety-provoking material,[56] a third investigation found a waiting-list no-treatment condition to be significantly inferior at post-therapy and follow-up to a CBT approach focused on teaching clients acceptance of uncertainty in life, more adaptive problem-solving orientations, exposure to catastrophic images underlying worrisome concerns, and correction of erroneous beliefs about worry.[57] Which of these several components, alone or in combination, were causative of improvement remains to be determined in future research.

Summary and conclusion

Considerable knowledge about the nature and functions of worry and GAD has been acquired over the past two decades. Current cognitive-behavioral therapies which incorporate relaxation training, cognitive therapy, and imagery rehearsals of somatic and cognitive coping responses to incipient anxiety have been shown in clinical trials to yield significant and maintained improvement in comparison to no-treatment, nonspecific, and some component control conditions. Because only 50% of clients so treated are returned to normal functioning, further treatment developments are necessary. New therapeutic elements, based on recent empirical findings and incorporated into existing cognitive-behavioral methods, include interpersonal psychotherapy, techniques from mindfulness/acceptance therapeutic orientations, acceptance of uncertainty, modification of erroneous beliefs about worry, and imagery exposure to catastrophic fears underlying worry. Hopefully, these and other directions will soon yield effective interventions for more people suffering from GAD.

Acknowledgement

Preparation of this chapter was supported in part by National Institute of Mental Health Research Grant MH-39172.

References

1. Freeston MH, Dugas MJ, Ladouceur R, Thoughts, images, worry, and anxiety, *Cognitive Ther Res* (1996) 20:265–73.

2. Rapee RM, The utilization of working memory by worry, *Behav Res Ther* (1993) 31:617–20.

3. Borkovec TD, Ray W, Stöber J, Worry: A cognitive phenomenon intimately linked to affective, physiological, and interpersonal behavioral processes, *Cognitive Ther Res* (1998) 22:561–76.

4. Borkovec TD, Inz J, The nature of worry in generalized anxiety disorder: A predominance of thought activity, *Behav Res Ther* (1990) 28:153–8.

5. Stöber J, Worry, problem elaboration, and suppression of imagery: The role of concreteness, *Behav Res Ther* (1998) 36: 751–6.

6. Stöber J, Borkovec TD, Reduced concreteness of worry in generalized anxiety disorder: Findings from a therapy study, *Cognitive Ther Res* (2002) 26:89–96.

7. Vrana SR, Cuthbert BN, Lang PJ, Fear imagery and text processing, *Psychophysiology* (1986) 23:247–53.

8. Borkovec TD, Robinson E, Pruzinsky T, DePree JA, Preliminary exploration of worry: Some characteristics and processes, *Behav Res Ther* (1983) 21:9–16.

9. Thayer JF, Friedman BH, Borkovec TD, Johnsen BH, Molina S, Phasic heart period reactions to cued threat and non-threat stimuli in generalized anxiety disorder, *Psychophysiology* (2000) 37:361–8.

10. Dugas MJ, Gagnon F, Ladouceur R, Freeston MH, Generalized anxiety disorder: A preliminary test of a conceptual model, *Behav Res Ther* (1998) 36:215–26.

11. MacLeod C, Information processing approaches to generalized anxiety disorder: Assessing the selective functioning of attention, interpretation, and memory in GAD patients. In: Heimberg RG, Turk CL, Mennin DS, eds, *Generalized anxiety disorder: Advances in research and practice.* (Guilford Press: New York, in press)

12. MacLeod C, Mathews A, Tata P, Attentional bias in emotional disorders, *J Abnorm Psychol* (1986) 95:15–20.

13. Horenstein M, Segui J, Chronometrics of attentional processes in anxiety disorders, *Psychopathology* (1997) 30:25–35.

14. Wenzel A, Holt CS, Dot probe performance in two specific phobias, *Br J Clin Psychol* (1999) 38:407–10.

15. Tata PR, Leibowitz JA, Prunty MJ, Cameron M, Attentional bias in obsessional compulsive disorder, *Behav Res Ther* (1996) 34:53–60.

16. MacLeod C, Mathews A, Anxiety and the allocation of attention to threat, *Quart J Exper Psychol* (1988) 40:653–70.

17. Mogg K, Bradley BP, Miller T, Potts H, Interpretation of homophones related to threat: Anxiety or response bias effects?, *Cognitive Ther Res* (1994) 18:461–77.

18. Clark DM, Salkovskis PM, Öst LG, et al., Misinterpretation of body sensations in panic disorder, *J Consult Clin Psychol* (1997) 65: 203–13.

19. Burke M, Mathews A, Autobiographical memory and clinical anxiety, *Cognition and Emotion* (1992) 6:23–35.

20. Becker ES, Roth WT, Andrich M, Margraf J, Explicit memory in anxiety disorders, *J Abnorm Psychol* (1999) 108:153–63.

21. Mogg K, Gardiner JM, Stavrous A, Golombok S, Recollective experience and recognition memory for threat in clinical anxiety states, *Bull Psychonomic Soc* (1992) 30:109–12.

22. Friedman B, Thayer J, Borkovec TD, Explicit memory bias for threat words in generalized anxiety disorder, *Behavior Therapy* (2000) 31:745–56.

23. Watts FN, Cognitive processing in phobias, *Behav Psychotherapy* (1986) 14:295–301.

24. Radomsky AS, Rachman S, Memory bias in obsessive-compulsive disorder (OCD), *Behav Res Ther* (1999) 37:605–18.

25. Vrana SR, Roodman A, Beckham JC, Selective processing of trauma-relevant words in posttraumatic stress disorder, *J Anxiety Disord* (1995) 9:515–30.

26. Mathews A, Mogg K, May J, Eysenck M, Implicit and explicit memory bias in anxiety, *J Abnorm Psychol* (1989) 98:236–40.

27. Becker ES, Rinck M, Roth WT, Margraf J, Don't worry and beware of white bears: Thought suppression in anxiety patients, *J Anxiety Res* (1998) 12:39–55.

28. Mathews A, Mogg K, Kentish J, Eysenck M, Effect of psychological treatment on cognitive bias in generalized anxiety disorder, *Behav Res Ther* (1995) 33:293–303.

29. Golombok S, Stavrou A, Bonn J, Mogg K, The effects of diazepam on anxiety-related cognitions, *Cognitive Ther Res* (1991) 15:459–67.

30. Mathews A, Mackintosh B, Induced emotional interpretation bias and anxiety, *J Abnorm Psychol* (2000) 109:602–15.

31. Hoehn-Saric R, McLeod DR, Zimmerli WD, Somatic manifestations in women with generalized anxiety disorder: Physiological responses to psychological stress, *Arch Gen Psychiatry* (1989) 46:1113–9.

32. Thayer JF, Friedman BH, Borkovec TD, Autonomic characteristics of generalized anxiety disorder and worry, *Biol Psychiatry* (1996) 39:255–66.

33. Marten PA, Brown TA, Barlow DH, Borkovec TD, Shear MK, Lydiard RB, Evaluation of the ratings comprising the associated symptom criterion of DSM-III-R generalized anxiety disorder, *J Nerv Ment Dis* (1993) 181:676–82.

34. Joormann J, Stöber J, Somatic symptoms of generalized anxiety disorder for the DSM-IV: Associations with pathological worry and depression symptoms in a nonclinical sample, *J Anxiety Disord* (1999) 13:491–503.

35. Borkovec TD, Hazlett-Stevens H, Diaz ML, The role of positive beliefs about worry in generalized anxiety disorder and its treatment, *Clin Psychol Psychotherapy* (1999) 6:126–38.

36. Grossman P, Stemmler G, Meinhardt E, Paced respiratory sinus arrythmia as an index of cardiac parasympathetic tone during varying behavioral tasks, *Psychophysiology* (1990) 27:404–16.

37. Metzger RL, Miller ML, Cohen M, Sofka M, Borkovec TD, Worry changes decision making: The effect of negative thoughts on cognitive processing, *J Clin Psychol* (1990) 46:78–88.

38. Porges SW, Autonomic regulation and attention. In: Campbell BA, Hayne H, Richardson R, eds, *Attention and information processing in infants and adults* (Erbaum: Hillside, NJ, 1992) 201–23.

39. Friedman BH, Thayer JF, Borkovec TD, Tyrrell RA, Johnson BH, Colombo R, Autonomic characteristics of nonclinical panic and blood phobia, *Biol Psychiatry* (1993) 34:298–310.

40. Roemer L, Molina S, Borkovec TD, The nature of generalized anxiety disorder: Worry content, *J Nerv Ment Dis* (1997) 185:314–9.

41. Butler G, Fennell M, Robson P, Gelder M, Comparison of behavior therapy and cognitive behavior therapy in the treatment of generalized anxiety disorder, *J Consult Clin Psychol* (1991) 59:167–75.

42 Schut AJ, Castonguay LG, Borkovec TD, Compulsive checking behaviors in generalized anxiety disorder, *J Clin Psychol* (2001) 57:705–15.

43. McGuire WJ, McGuire CV, The content, structure, and operation of thought systems. In: Wyer RS, Srull TK, eds, *Advances in social cognition* (Erlbaum: Hillside, NJ, 1991) 1–78.

44. Borkovec TD, Alcaine O, Behar E, Avoidance theory of worry and generalized anxiety disorder. In: Heimberg RG, Turk CL, Mennin DS, eds, *Generalized anxiety disorder: Advances in research and practice* (Guilford Press: New York, in press)

45. Chambless DL, Gillis MM, Cognitive therapy of anxiety disorders, *J Consult Clin Psychol* (1993) 61:248–60.

46. Borkovec TD, Ruscio A, Psychotherapy for generalized anxiety disorder, *J Clin Psychiatry* (2001) 62(suppl 11): 37–42.

47. Borkovec TD, Whisman MA, Psychological treatment for generalized anxiety disorder. In: Mavissakalian MR, Prien RF, eds, *Long-term treatments of anxiety disorders*. (American Psychiatric Association: Washington, DC, 1996) 171–99.

48. Öst LG, Breitholz E, Applied relaxation vs. cognitive therapy in the treatment of generalized anxiety disorder, *Behav Res Ther* (2000) 8:777–90.

49. Borkovec TD, Newman MG, Pincus A, Lytle R, A component analysis of cognitive behavioral therapy for generalized anxiety disorder and the role of interpersonal problems, *J Consult Clin Psychol* (2002) 70:288–98.

50. Newman MG, Castonguay LG, Borkovec TD, Molnar C, Integrative therapy for generalized anxiety disorder. In: Heimberg RG, Turk CL, Mennin DS, eds, *Generalized anxiety disorder: Advances in research and practice*. (Guilford Press: New York, in press).

51. Roemer L, Orsillo SM, Expanding our conceptualization of and treatment for generalized anxiety disorder: Integrating mindfulness/acceptance-based approaches with existing cognitive-behavioral models, *Clin Psychol: Science and Practice* (2002) 9: 54–68.

52. Kabat-Zinn J, Massion AO, Kristeller J, et al., Effectiveness of a meditation-based stress reduction program in the treatment of anxiety disorders, *Am J Psychiatry* (1992) 149:936–43.

53. Dugas MJ, Freeston MH, Ladouceur R, Intolerance of uncertainty and problem orientation in worry, *Cognitive Ther Res* (1997) 21:593–606.

54. Ladouceur R, Dugas MJ, Freeston MH, Rheaume, J, Blais F, Boisvert JM, Gagnon F, Thibodeau N, Specificity of generalized anxiety disorder symptoms and processes, *Behavior Therapy* (1999) 30:191–207.

55. Wells A, A metacognitive model and therapy for generalized anxiety disorder, *Clin Psychol Psychotherapy* 6: 86–95.

56. Craske MG, *Anxiety disorders: Psychological approaches to theory and treatment* (Westview Press: Boulder, CO, 1999).

57. Ladouceur R, Dugas MJ, Freeston MH, Leger E, Gagnon F, Thibodeau N, Efficacy of cognitive-behavioral treatment for generalized anxiety disorder: Evaluation in a controlled clinical trial, *J Consult Clin Psychol* (2000) 68:957–64.

9

Treatment of Generalized Anxiety Disorder: Do Benzodiazepines Still Have A Role?

Gretchen Carlson and Peter P Roy-Byrne

Generalized anxiety disorder (GAD) is a prevalent, chronic, and disabling condition.[1] Although GAD was initially defined as a disorder in the DSM-III in 1980, at first it was incompletely accepted as a distinct Axis I disorder (see Chapter 1), perhaps because of its brief duration, requirement for only mild impairment, and strong comorbidity with depression. Some viewed GAD as a personality style or vulnerability trait that predisposed to major depression, or even as an indicator of severity of major depression.[2] In cases of GAD with comorbid depression, it was unclear whether GAD alone led to impairment, or whether the impairment associated with GAD could be attributed to major depression. Although two small primary care studies[3,4] found that disability in pure major depressive disorder (MDD) was greater than that in GAD, large population studies (see also Chapter 2) have found comparable disability in pure MDD and GAD. Given the longer duration and greater degree of impairment associated with DSM-IV GAD, there is no question that more aggressive treatment is warranted. The question then becomes how best to treat GAD, with the goal of alleviating the broad range of symptoms, while minimizing liability and side effects associated with the treatment.

Since the introduction of benzodiazepines in the 1950s, GAD has been treated primarily with this class of medications. Despite a number of known disadvantages, such as abuse, withdrawal syndromes, disinhibition and cognitive impairment, benzodiazepines were found to be highly efficacious, with a superior therapeutic index to previously used hypnotic agents. One drawback of benzodiazepines, however, is that they do not treat, and may worsen, comorbid major depression that occurs in up to two-thirds of cases of GAD.[5] This fact was poorly appreciated by many clinicians, especially those in primary care. In the past decade, antidepressants have been found to be equally or more efficacious in the treatment of GAD.[6] These developments demand a reassessment of the role of benzodiazepines in the treatment of GAD. With this in mind, we will review evidence for the efficacy of this class of medications compared with other pharmacologic and psychotherapeutic treatments of GAD; summarize the current state of knowledge concerning side effects and risks; and finally arrive at an assessment of the likely future role of this class of medications for GAD.

Benefits of benzodiazepines

Studies of benzodiazepines vs psychotherapy in GAD

Numerous double-blind placebo-controlled studies have shown benzodiazepines to be efficacious in the treatment of GAD, with greatest evidence from recent studies focusing on DSM-III-R and DSM-IV definitions of the disorder. Failure to find positive effects in earlier studies of benzodiazepines may be related to their selection of cases using DSM-II equivalent and DSM-III GAD, with inherent poor reliability and lower severity respectively. For example, Solomon and Hart[7] reviewed 78 double-blind placebo-controlled studies and found that benzodiazepines were not more efficacious than placebo in the treatment of 'neurotic anxiety', an ill-defined nosologic category. Barlow[8] reviewed eight double-blind placebo-controlled studies using the Hamilton anxiety rating scale (HAM-A) as outcome and found similar reductions in HAM-A in both placebo and treatment groups, probably because of the brief one-month duration of GAD and the likelihood that spontaneous remission caused high placebo response rates. Nonetheless, the dropout rates in the placebo groups were higher in five of the six studies reporting this data, suggesting greater efficacy in the benzodiazepine group. Consistent with the above explanations for negative findings, Shapiro[9]

found that diazepam was more effective than placebo in the treatment of severe GAD.

In studies of DSM-III-R and DSM-IV GAD, benzodiazepines have been superior to placebo in the acute treatment of symptoms in most studies.[6,10] Approximately two-thirds of patients with GAD get some benefit from benzodiazepines. They work quickly, with therapeutic onset in the first 1–2 weeks of treatment. GAD patients require approximately half the dose of benzodiazepines as those with panic disorder. Benzodiazepines are especially effective for the treatment of somatic anxiety, whereas antidepressants are more effective in the treatment of psychic anxiety.[10] However, patients with comorbid depressive symptoms do not respond as well to benzodiazepines as those without depression.[6]

The efficacy of benzodiazepines in the long-term treatment of GAD is less clear, since only a few studies have examined this issue. In a six-month open trial, clorazepate showed continued efficacy with no evidence of tolerance to anxiolytic effects.[11] In a 16-week placebo-controlled study, lorazepam and alprazolam also showed continued efficacy over placebo.[12] While, in an 8-week placebo-controlled study, lorazepam showed improvement superior to placebo after 6 but not 8 weeks,[13] this study was a multicenter trial, and in trials of this kind recruitment of heterogeneous patients and poor control of diagnostic procedures can confound results.

Studies of benzodiazepines vs. other medications in GAD

Double-blind studies have proven buspirone to be as efficacious as diazepam, lorazepam, clorazepate, and alprazolam in the acute treatment of GAD.[11,14–22] Therapeutic effects are delayed 2–4 weeks with buspirone.

Suggestions that buspirone results in more sustained clinical improvement than benzodiazepines is based on a single, 6-week controlled trial of 120 GAD patients[22] in which buspirone, lorazepam, and placebo were all discontinued, followed by a 4-week placebo phase to assess duration of clinical response. The increase in anxiety symptoms in the lorazepam group was most likely due to withdrawal or rapid loss of therapeutic effect (mirroring the rapid onset of benzodiazepine effect), while sustained 'response' in buspirone-treated patients may have represented only slower offset of therapeutic effect (mirroring its slower onset of effect). Unlike benzodiazepines, buspirone appears to have greater effect on psychic anxiety than somatic symptoms. It is not associated with tolerance or withdrawal symptoms, and it does not cause sedation.

Patients who have been treated long-term with benzodiazepines tend not to respond well when switched to buspirone. DeMartinis et al.[23] compared 735 patients with GAD who were treated with benzodiazepines, buspirone, or placebo. They found that clinical response was similar in those on buspirone and benzodiazepines if there was no prior history of treatment with benzodiazepines or treatment with benzodiazepines had been discontinued more than one month prior to treatment with buspirone. In those treated with benzodiazepines within one month of starting buspirone, there was less clinical improvement and greater drop-out rates due to lack of efficacy. These results may indicate that prior benzodiazepine treatment sensitizes patients to expect rapid and subjectively easy to detect anxiolysis. Alternatively, it may be that previous treatment with benzodiazepines is a 'marker' for greater illness severity. In a double-blind trial[24] of 44 patients with GAD treated with lorazepam for 5 weeks and then randomized to buspirone or placebo during a 2-week lorazepam taper, buspirone was superior to placebo in decreasing anxiety symptoms during benzodiazepine withdrawal. But due to the short duration of prior treatment, this does not obviate the above explanations.

Benzodiazepines have been compared to antidepressants in a number of double-blind studies. Kahn et al.[25] compared imipramine to chlordiazepoxide in GAD patients without comorbid depression and found that imipramine was better at treating psychic anxiety symptoms, whereas alprazolam was more effective in the treatment of somatic symptoms. In a comparison of imipramine, trazodone, diazepam, and placebo in the treatment of 230 patients with GAD,[6] diazepam showed the greatest reduction in anxiety in the first 2 weeks, while imipramine was superior for the remainder of the 8-week study, with 73% response for imipramine, 69% for trazodone, 66% for diazepam, and 47% for placebo. Similar results were found in a comparison of imipramine, paroxetine, and 2′-chlordesmethyldiazepam in 81 patients with GAD.[28] 2′-chlordesmethyldiazepam showed early improvement, while the antidepressants resulted in the greatest improvement at the end of the trial. Again, the antidepressants showed greater efficacy in treating psychic symptoms, and the benzodiazepine resulted in greater improvement in somatic complaints.[10]

Studies of psychotherapy vs. benzodiazepines in GAD

Although a review of several reports has suggested that the use of benzodiazepines in combination with psychotherapy as a treatment for GAD is theoretically problematic for a number of reasons,[27] there is little evidence supporting this contention. Benzodiazepines could interfere with psychotherapy through anterograde amnesia, but this has not been seen, perhaps because at therapeutic doses clinically significant cognitive impairment would be less likely to occur. While the use of benzodiazepines might induce state-dependent learning, leading to decreased retention once benzodiazepines are discontinued, this is unlikely to occur with clinically prescribed doses. While benzodiazepines also may interfere with habituation during exposure therapy, earlier studies[28] have failed to demonstrate that this occurs in phobic patients undergoing desensitization. By lowering anxiety, benzodiazepines may decrease motivation to participate in therapy, although, in this case, therapy would no longer be necessary. Benzodiazepines also function much like avoidance strategies, and may encourage further use of maladaptive avoidance that may prolong symptoms.[29]

Three clinical trials have compared psychotherapy and benzodiazepine treatments used independently. As expected, benzodiazepines result in earlier relief followed by relapse of symptoms at discontinuation, whereas psychotherapy leads to more sustained response. Lindsay et al.[30] randomized 40 patients with DSM-III GAD to a one-month course of cognitive-behavioral therapy (CBT), anxiety management training (AMT), lorazepam, or a wait-list control group. Patients in the psychotherapy groups received 2 sessions per week, and patients in the lorazepam group took 1 mg TID for 10 days, then 1 mg BID for 10 days, and then 1 mg prn for the final 10 days. The benzodiazepine group showed the earliest and greatest improvement, but this effect decreased as the taper progressed, and by the end of the study the benzodiazepine group was not significantly less anxious than the placebo group. The psychotherapy groups showed significant improvement starting at week 3, but were not significantly different from each other. At the 3-month follow-up, the psychotherapy groups showed maintenance of treatment gains, but more than 50% of the lorazepam group had resumed treatment due to lack of sustained effect after discontinuation. This study does not really mirror the benzodiazepine regimen that would be prescribed for most GAD patients (i.e. continuous low dose use would be more typical than intermittent prn use after brief continuous use).

Power et al.[31,32] conducted two studies comparing psychotherapy and benzodiazepines. The first study[31] was a 9-week placebo-controlled trial of 31 patients who met DSM-III criteria for GAD, who were randomized to CBT, diazepam, or placebo. CBT appeared superior to placebo and diazepam at the end of the study, based on patient self-report and overall assessment of the practitioner. However, there were large within-group variations in response to the treatments, and the investigators were not blinded to who was assigned to the CBT group.

In their second study, Power et al.[32] assigned 101 patients with one-month history of GAD symptoms to one of five groups: diazepam alone, CBT alone, placebo, CBT plus diazepam, or CBT plus placebo. This study took place in a primary care setting over 10 weeks with a 6-month follow-up. Those assigned to CBT received a maximum of 7 sessions over 9 weeks, while the diazepam groups received placebo for the first week, then 5 mg TID for 6 weeks, then 5 mg BID for one week, 5 mg QHS for one week, and finally placebo for the last week. The outcomes measured were severity of symptoms and overall change. At the end of treatment, the greatest improvement in both outcomes occurred in the CBT plus diazepam group, but the results were not significantly different from CBT alone or CBT plus placebo. Diazepam alone was not better than placebo. At 6-month follow-up, those individuals who had received CBT alone or in combination with diazepam or placebo had lower referral rates than those treated with diazepam or placebo alone. This suggests that CBT has a more sustained treatment gain whether combined with medication or not, and also suggests that diazepam, at this therapeutic dose, did not adversely interfere with CBT effects.

In contrast to these studies, similar studies in patients with panic disorder suggest that CBT has a worse outcome in those treated concurrently with benzodiazepines if the patients attribute their improvement to the medication.[33] A detrimental outcome was associated particularly with high-potency benzodiazepines, whereas low-potency benzodiazepines and antidepressants appeared to have no effect.[34]

In a recent meta-analysis of controlled trials of CBT and pharmacotherapy that included 23 benzodiazepine treatment interventions and 22 CBT interventions, Gould et al.[35] found that the effect size for benzodiazepines (0.7) was comparable to that of CBT (0.7). Although this was not a direct comparison, it is consistent with earlier results that suggest that the two interventions are equally efficacious in alleviating anxiety symptoms during ongoing treatment. CBT had significantly greater effects on comorbid depressive symptoms based on the three studies that included depressive measures. CBT also showed greater maintenance of treatment gains.

Summary

On balance, the available evidence reviewed above clearly indicates that benzodiazepines are efficacious for more rigorously and recently defined (and more clinically severe) GAD. However, there is no evidence that they are more effective than antidepressants or buspirone, and there are some inconsistent suggestions that they may be inferior in some ways. Psychotherapy appears to measure up fairly well, and may have more long-term sustainability than pharmacotherapy. The major and only obvious advantage of benzodiazepines is that they act quite rapidly, a unique effect. They are not effective against depressive symptoms and may even aggravate them. Their previously noted advantage of being more tolerable than older antidepressants is not as true today, although they may still be more tolerable for some patients with bothersome selective serotonin reuptake inhibitor (SSRI) side effects (e.g. sexual dysfunction).

Risks of benzodiazepines

Dependence and discontinuation

One of the primary concerns in prescribing benzodiazepines for any disorder is the risk of dependence and withdrawal.[36,37] Discontinuation of benzodiazepines after long-term use often results in increased anxiety. This anxiety may be due to withdrawal symptoms secondary to rebound loss of GABA-mediated neuronal inhibition; to a return of the original anxiety disorder that is no longer being treated; or to a combination of the two, often termed 'rebound' anxiety (relapse made worse by withdrawal). Although these three possibilities are difficult to distinguish clinically, and there may be considerable overlap in symptoms, the nature and severity of the underlying disorder always contributes in a major way. For example, after treatment with diazepam for 6 weeks, GAD patients experienced increased anxiety with discontinuation of diazepam, while non-anxious volunteers did not experience anxiety after discontinuation.[38] Similarly, compared to patients with panic disorder, patients with GAD tend to have less severe discontinuation symptoms.[39]

Increased risk of difficult discontinuation has been associated with a number of factors which need to be considered in the risk-benefit analysis in choosing treatment for patients with GAD. In addition to the underlying severity of anxiety, well-studied patient-related factors include: a history of substance abuse, particularly alcoholism; a family history of substance abuse; and personality traits of passivity, dependency, resourcelessness, childishness, and submissiveness.[40–42] Preliminary evidence also suggests the importance of ongoing psychosocial stress and attitude toward treatment.[43,44] Because people suffering from GAD use worrying as a coping strategy,[45] patients experiencing high psychosocial stressors at the time of discontinuation may be at greater risk for increased worry and anxiety symptoms due to deficits in problem-solving and coping skills. In support of this theory, O'Connor et al.[46] found that an increase in severity of discontinuation symptoms has been associated with lower education level and lower quality of life. In panic disorder, attitude toward the medication may also influence discontinuation symptoms, with greater difficulty associated with belief that improvement is due only to medication rather than to patients' own efforts in therapy.[33] This may explain why CBT has increased successful discontinuation of benzodiazepines in panic disorder patients,[47] though this strategy has yet to be tested in patients with GAD.

A number of treatment-related factors may also worsen discontinuation severity. These include longer duration of benzodiazepine use (greater than 6 months);[11,36,48] prior use, high potency,[49] dose, and rate of taper (decreasing the dose by 25% every 3 days will produce some, but not severe, symptoms in most patients); shorter half-life (if rate of taper is abrupt) and dosing regimen (an as-needed dosing regimen may reinforce pill-taking due to the mild withdrawal or rebound symptoms that may occur with intermittent use).

Although there is clearly a potential for increased anxiety with discontinuation of benzodiazepines, these symptoms appear to be amenable to clinical management. While use of agents that do not primarily treat the underlying anxiety syndrome has been only modestly effective (i.e. beta blockers, which attenuate autonomic but not psychological withdrawal symptoms; carbamazepine, which modestly affects discontinuation in panic but not GAD patients;[39] and valproate, which curiously had no effect despite similarities to carbamazepine[50]), antidepressants or buspirone may be more effective.[51] Rickels et al. examined success at a 4–6 week tapered discontinuation in a double-blind placebo-controlled trial using 4 weeks of imipramine or buspirone pretreatment in 107 GAD patients who were long-term benzodiazepine users. Only those in the imipramine group were significantly more successful at discontinuing benzodiazepines than placebo, while those in the buspirone group were nonsignificantly better than placebo. However, in a double-blind placebo-controlled trial of 44 patients with GAD who were being discontinued from lorazepam,[24] buspirone was significantly better than placebo in decreasing withdrawal symptoms and rebound anxiety. Curiously, these results were not replicated with a different, albeit poorly designed, study using paroxetine.[52]

Finally, two studies have examined the use of CBT for benzodiazepine discontinuation in patients with panic disorder. Findings suggest that CBT can improve success rates and result in less benzodiazepine use in the follow-up period. Otto et al.[47] found that 76% of patients who received CBT versus 25% who had not received CBT successfully tapered off benzodiazepines. Spiegel et al.[53] found no difference in discontinuation rates between those who did and did not receive CBT, but at the 6-month follow-up, half of the subjects who had discontinued benzodiazepines without CBT were again receiving benzodiazepines, while no subjects in the CBT group had resumed benzodiazepine use.

Abuse

Dose escalation is rare in GAD patients who do not have a history of abuse. Rickels et al.[54] found no increase in dose in 119 GAD patients on benzodiazepines for an average of 8 years, nor were there any other signs of abuse. Indeed, the majority of evidence suggests that benzodiazepine abuse mostly occurs in the context of other substance abuse, particularly opiate dependence, but also alcoholism. This is corroborated by data from animal studies that show that benzodiazepines are not self-administered by animals that are naïve to sedatives,[55] with inconsistent results in studies of animals with previous exposure to sedatives.[56,57] The suggestion that there is a small number of patients that abuse solely benzodiazepines has never been substantiated by a descriptive study of the characteristics of these patients or confirmation that they are not abusing, or have not abused in the past, other substances.[58]

Studies that have documented 'preference' for benzodiazepines in certain non-abusing populations, usually social drinkers or anxious individuals, have been used to suggest that these patients may be at greater risk for abuse. However, such paradigms may only measure patients' experience with sedative hypnotic drugs, with their choice or preference indicating recognition or familiarity as much as abuse liability.[59,60] Long-term benzodiazepine use does not appear to be a gateway for abuse of other substances.[61]

Some studies suggest that alcoholics do respond differently to benzodiazepines.[62–65] When benzodiazepines were administered to alcoholics and non-alcoholics, EEG activity was different in the alcoholic group.[62] In addition, imaging and postmortem studies show changes in benzodiazepine receptors and low cortical GABA levels in alcoholics.[63–65] Hence, the clinically observed increased risk of abuse in patients with alcohol or other substance abuse disorders may have a biological basis. This group also shows a preference for certain kinds of benzodiazepines, particularly alprazolam, diazepam, and lorazepam over clorazepate, chlordiazepoxide, and oxazepam.[66] When treatment with benzodiazepines is necessary in alcoholics, using the latter benzodiazepines may decrease potential for abuse.

But the clinical lore that prior substance-abusing patients should never be given benzodiazepines, even if they have been recovered for some time, is now being questioned by experts in the field.[58] The risk of abuse appears to remain high in patients with severe alcohol dependence, polysubstance dependence, and antisocial personality disorder.[58] Yet for patients with mild to moderate alcohol problems, there is no rationale for not treating with benzodiazepines, with some caveats: clearly, other alternatives, such as antidepressants and psychotherapy, should be tried first; confirmation of ongoing recovery from alcoholism should be obtained; provision of a limited amount of medication with close monitoring is essential; a single provider should be dispensing; and tapering should be attempted periodically.[58]

Cognitive impairment

Benzodiazepines are known to cause anterograde amnesia, i.e. impairment in the ability to form long-term memories.[67–69] Short-term retrograde and procedural memory, which are required to learn new skills, are not affected by benzodiazepines.[70,71] Therefore, someone taking a benzodiazepine could learn a new skill, such as how to use a computer, but may not recall that he learned it. Benzodiazepines may also cause a transient global amnesia, an episode in which the patient appears to be functioning normally but has no recall of that period of time afterwards.[72,73]

Although some studies have found a correlation between amnesia and sedation,[70,74,75] the risk of amnesia continues in the chronic user despite development of tolerance to the sedation.[71,76] All benzodiazepines have the ability to cause anterograde amnesia, but high-potency benzodiazepines cause amnesia more often.[72] The half-life of the drug does not appear to affect the likelihood of amnesia. Cognitive impairment with benzodiazepines is more likely with higher dose, older age, and increasing task difficulty. The elderly are more vulnerable to the amnestic effects of benzodiazepines, and memory impairment is more prolonged in this population.[77] Alcohol increases the risk of anterograde amnesia when used concurrently with benzodiazepines by affecting the chloride ion channels on the benzodiazepine receptors.[78] In addition, any medication with anticholinergic properties, such as antidepressants, antipsychotics, antihistamines, and antiparkinsonian medications, may interact with benzodiazepines to increase amnesia.[79]

Several studies have looked at cognitive performance in long-term benzodiazepine users, during and after discontinuation. Most studies found no tolerance to amnestic effects in long-term users[80,81] with the exception of those taking Alprazolam XR.[82] While one study found persisting cognitive deficits after discontinuation in long-term users,[83] this study could not separate characteristics of the underlying illness prompting treatment from the effects of that treatment. Consistent with this, two other studies found that, following discontinuation, the cognitive impairment caused by benzodiazepines was reversible.[80,84] A corollary concern has been the possibility that long-term use might result in 'brain damage', initially suggested by studies reporting greater CT scan atrophy in some chronic users.[85,86] However, a more recent study that provided appropriate anxiety disorder control groups and controlled for medical confounds such as history of head injury or epilepsy clearly showed that such brain abnormalities do not occur as a consequence of long-term benzodiazepine use.[87]

Psychomotor impairment

In terms of psychomotor impairment, benzodiazepines increase the risk of falls in the elderly and may increase the risk of stress fractures, even at the low doses currently recommended for elderly patients.[88] Risk factors associated with falls include short half-life,[89,90] sudden increase in dose,[89] use of two or more benzodiazepines concurrently[89,91] or in conjunction with other psychotropics or antidiabetic agents, cognitive impairment, high comorbidity, age greater than 80 years, and hospitalization for more than 17 days.[90] However, evidence suggests that antidepressants produce an increase in falls comparable to benzodiazepines[92] and a recent study[93] showed that there was no difference in risk of fall between SSRIs and older, more sedating, antidepressants. Benzodiazepines also result in impaired driving performance and increased motor vehicle accidents in all age groups. In contrast to falls, driving impairment is more clearly associated with longer half-life for both acute and chronic benzodiazepine users. Furthermore, there is little evidence that newer antidepressants cause psychomotor impairment in younger patients.

Behavioral disinhibition

Behavioral disinhibition has been reported anecdotally with benzodiazepines. Disinhibition has been associated with higher doses of benzodiazepines and higher pretreatment hostility. Few placebo-controlled studies have been conducted on disinhibition with benzodiazepines. Rothschild et al.[94] compared the incidence of disinhibition, characterized by self-injurious acts, assaultive behavior, need for restraints or seclusion, need for greater staff observation, and decreased privileges, in 323 psychiatric inpatients who were taking alprazolam, clonazepam, or no benzodiazepines. They found no difference in frequency of disinhibition among these three groups. Overall, even in this high-risk population the rate of disinhibited behaviors was low. Although this may have been mainly due to the highly structured hospital environment, the results suggest that disinhibition would be a rare event in low-risk patients.

Summary

The evidence reviewed indicates that, while the benzodiazepines are clearly associated with abuse, dependence, cognitive and psychomotor impairment, and disinhibition, the clinical impact of these problems in GAD patients is modest at best. Abuse is unlikely to occur in patients without active substance abuse, and dependence, when it occurs in a proportion of patients, is both predictable and manageable.

Cognitive and psychomotor impairment is mostly problematic in the elderly, and in this group of patients antidepressants (particularly some of the older tricyclics) may pose similar risks. Despite the minimal nature of most of these risks, however, they supercede in most cases those of antidepressants, and obviously of CBT.

Do benzodiazepines offer something unique?

Clearly, benzodiazepines are an effective treatment for generalized anxiety disorder. This class of medications results in rapid relief of symptoms and is well tolerated by patients overall. Benzodiazepines' liability for dependence and discontinuation reactions can be managed reasonably well in most clinical settings. Their association with cognitive and psychomotor impairment, although not a problem that persists after discontinuation, creates a number of risks to optimal function, both for younger individuals with jobs that demand complex information processing, and for older individuals because of their increased sensitivity to cognitive impairment as well as their propensity for falls. Although these risks may not be generic or widespread, when they are combined with the growing evidence that antidepressants can treat GAD effectively, we must conclude that benzodiazepines are no longer the first-line treatment for GAD. However, they are still useful as adjuncts during the initial treatment of GAD, as augmenting agents for patients on antidepressants who still experience considerable somatic anxiety, and as a viable, second-line, long-term treatment for antidepressant and buspirone non-responders.

References

1. Wittchen HU, Hoyer J, Generalized anxiety disorder: nature and course, *J Clin Psychiatry* (2001) **62** (Suppl 11): 15–9; discussion 20–1.

2. Roy-Byrne PP, Katon W, Generalized anxiety disorder in primary care: the precursor/modifier pathway to increased health care utilization, *J Clin Psychiatry* (1997) **58 Suppl** 3: 34–8; discussion 9–40.

3. Olfson M, Fireman B, Weissman MM et al., Mental disorders and disability among patients in a primary care group practice, *Am J Psychiatry* (1997) **154**: 1734–40.

4. Schonfeld WH, Verboncoeur CJ, Fifer SK et al., The functioning and well-being of patients with unrecognized anxiety disorders and major depressive disorder, *J Affect Disord* (1997) **43**: 105–19.

5. Kessler RC, DuPont RL, Berglund P et al., Impairment in pure and comorbid generalized anxiety disorder and major depression at 12 months in two national surveys, *Am J Psychiatry* (1999) **156**: 1915–23.

6. Rickels K, Downing R, Schweizer E et al., Antidepressants for the treatment of generalized anxiety disorder. A placebo-controlled comparison of imipramine, trazodone, and diazepam, *Arch Gen Psychiatry* (1993) **50**: 884–95.

7. Solomon K, Hart R, Pitfalls and prospects in clinical research on antianxiety drugs: benzodiazepines and placebo—a research review, *J Clin Psychiatry* (1978) **39**: 823–31.

8. Barlow DH, *Anxiety and its disorders: the nature and treatment of anxiety and panic*, (New York: Guilford Press, 1988).

9. Shapiro AK, Struening EL, Shapiro E et al., Diazepam: how much better than placebo? *J Psychiatr Res* (1982) **17**: 51–73.

10. Hoehn-Saric R, McLeod DR, Zimmerli WD, Differential effects of alprazolam and imipramine in generalized anxiety disorder: somatic versus psychic symptoms, *J Clin Psychiatry* (1988) **49**: 293–301.

11. Rickels K, Schweizer E, Csanalosi I et al., Long-term treatment of anxiety and risk of withdrawal. Prospective comparison of clorazepate and buspirone, *Arch Gen Psychiatry* (1988) **45**: 444–50.

12. Cohn JB, Wilcox CS, Long-term comparison of alprazolam, lorazepam and placebo in patients with an anxiety disorder, *Pharmacotherapy* (1984) **4**: 93–8.

13. Cutler NR, Sramek JJ, Keppel Hesselink JM et al., A double-blind, placebo-controlled study comparing the efficacy and safety of ipsapirone versus lorazepam in patients with generalized anxiety disorder: a prospective multicenter trial, *J Clin Psychopharmacol* (1993) **13**: 429–37.

14. Ansseau M, Papart P, Gerard MA et al., Controlled comparison of buspirone and oxazepam in generalized anxiety, *Neuropsychobiology* (1990) **24**: 74–8.

15. Cohn JB, Bowden CL, Fisher JG et al., Double-blind comparison of buspirone and clorazepate in anxious outpatients, *Am J Med* (1986) **80**: 10–6.

16. Enkelmann R, Alprazolam versus buspirone in the treatment of outpatients with generalized anxiety disorder, *Psychopharmacology (Berl)* (1991) **105**: 428–32.

17. Feighner JP, Merideth CH, Hendrickson GA, A double-blind comparison of buspirone and diazepam in outpatients with generalized anxiety disorder, *J Clin Psychiatry* (1982) **43**: 103–8.

18. Murphy SM, Owen R, Tyrer P, Comparative assessment of efficacy and withdrawal symptoms after 6 and 12 weeks' treatment with diazepam or buspirone, *Br J Psychiatry* (1989) **154**: 529–34.

19. Petracca A, Nisita C, McNair D et al., Treatment of generalized anxiety disorder: preliminary clinical experience with buspirone, *J Clin Psychiatry* (1990) **51 Suppl**: 31–9.

20. Rickels K, Weisman K, Norstad N et al., Buspirone and diazepam in anxiety: a controlled study, *J Clin Psychiatry* (1982) **43**: 81–6.

21. Strand M, Hetta J, Rosen A et al., A double-blind, controlled trial in primary care patients with generalized anxiety: a comparison between buspirone and oxazepam, *J Clin Psychiatry* (1990) **51** (Suppl): 40–5.

22. Laakmann G, Schule C, Lorkowski G et al., Buspirone and lorazepam in the treatment of generalized anxiety disorder in outpatients, *Psychopharmacology (Berl)* (1998) **136**: 357–66.

23. DeMartinis N, Rynn M, Rickels K et al., Prior benzodiazepine use and buspirone response in the treatment of generalized anxiety disorder, *J Clin Psychiatry* (2000) **61**: 91–4.

24. Delle Chiaie R, Pancheri P, Casacchia M et al., Assessment of the efficacy of buspirone in patients affected by generalized anxiety disorder, shifting to buspirone from prior treatment with lorazepam: a

placebo-controlled, double-blind study, *J Clin Psychopharmacol* (1995) **15**: 12–19.

25. Kahn RJ, McNair DM, Lipman RS et al., Imipramine and chlordiazepoxide in depressive and anxiety disorders. II. Efficacy in anxious outpatients, *Arch Gen Psychiatry* (1986) **43**: 79–85.

26. Rocca P, Fonzo V, Scotta M et al., Paroxetine efficacy in the treatment of generalized anxiety disorder, *Acta Psychiatr Scand* (1997) **95**: 444–50.

27. Wardle J, Behaviour therapy and benzodiazepines: allies or antagonists? *Br J Psychiatry* (1990) **156**: 163–8.

28. Hafner J, Marks I, Exposure in vivo of agoraphobics: contributions of diazepam, group exposure, and anxiety evocation, *Psychol Med* (1976) **6**: 71–88.

29. Person JB MD, Tucker DE, Common misconceptions about the nature and treatment of generalized anxiety disorder, *Psychiatric Annals* (2001) **31**: 501–7.

30. Lindsay WR, Gamsu CV, McLaughlin E et al., A controlled trial of treatments for generalized anxiety, *Br J Clin Psychol* (1987) **26** (Pt 1): 3–15.

31. Power KG, Jerrom DW, Simpson RJ, Mitchell, MJ, et al., A controlled comparison of cognitive-behaviour therapy, diazepam, and placebo in the management of generalised anxiety, *Behav Psychother* (1989) **17**: 1–14.

32. Power KG, Simpson RJ, Swanson V et al., Controlled comparison of pharmacological and psychological treatment of generalized anxiety disorder in primary care, *Br J Gen Pract* (1990) **40**: 289–94.

33. Basoglu M, Marks IM, Kilic C et al., Alprazolam and exposure for panic disorder with agoraphobia. Attribution of improvement to medication predicts subsequent relapse, *Br J Psychiatry* (1994) **164**: 652–9.

34. Westra HA, Stewart SH, Cognitive behavioural therapy and pharmacotherapy: complementary or contradictory approaches to the treatment of anxiety? *Clin Psychol Rev* (1998) **18**: 307–40.

35. Gould RA OM, Pollack MH, Yap L, Cognitive behavioral and pharmacologic treatment of generalized anxiety disorder: A preliminary meta-analysis, *Behav Therapy* (1997) **28**: 285–305.

36. Rickels K, Schweizer E, Case WG et al., Long-term therapeutic use of benzodiazepines. I. Effects of abrupt discontinuation, *Arch Gen Psychiatry* (1990) **47**: 899–907.

37. Rickels K, Schweizer E, The spectrum of generalised anxiety in clinical practice: the role of short-term, intermittent treatment, *Br J Psychiatry* (Suppl) (1998): 49–54.

38. Pourmotabbed T, McLeod DR, Hoehn-Saric R et al., Treatment, discontinuation, and psychomotor effects of diazepam in women with generalized anxiety disorder, *J Clin Psychopharmacol* (1996) **16**: 202–7.

39. Klein E, Colin V, Stolk J et al., Alprazolam withdrawal in patients with panic disorder and generalized anxiety disorder: vulnerability and effect of carbamazepine, *Am J Psychiatry* (1994) **151**: 1760–6.

40. Tyrer P, Owen R, Dawling S, Gradual withdrawal of diazepam after long-term therapy, *Lancet* (1983) **1**: 1402–6.

41. Rickels K, Schweizer E, Case GW et al., Benzodiazepine dependence, withdrawal severity, and clinical outcome: effects of personality, *Psychopharmacol Bull* (1988) **24**: 415–20.

42. Schweizer E, Rickels K, DeMartinis N et al., The effect of personality on withdrawal severity and taper outcome in benzodiazepine dependent patients, *Psychol Med* (1998) **28**: 713–20.

43. Gray JA, Davis N, Feldon J et al., Animal models of anxiety, *Prog Neuropsychopharmacol* (1981) **5**: 143–57.

44. Davidson TL, Lucki I, The long-term effects of diazepam and pentylenetetrazol on behavioral sensitivity to a stressor, *Pharmacol Biochem Behav* (1987) **27**: 99–103.

45. Wells A, A cognitive model of generalized anxiety disorder, *Behav Modif* (1999) **23**: 526–55.

46. O'Connor K, Belanger L, Marchand A et al., Psychological distress and adaptational problems associated with discontinuation of benzodiazepines, *Addict Behav* (1999) **24**: 537–41.

47. Otto MW, Pollack MH, Sachs GS et al., Discontinuation of benzodiazepine treatment: efficacy of cognitive-behavioral therapy for patients with panic disorder, *Am J Psychiatry* (1993) **150**: 1485-90.

48. Rickels K, Freeman EW, Prior benzodiazepine exposure and benzodiazepine treatment outcome, *J Clin Psychiatry* (2000) **61**: 409–13.

49. Tyrer P, Dependence as a limiting factor in the clinical use of minor tranquillizers, *Pharmacol Ther* (1988) **36**: 173–88.

50. Rickels K, Schweizer E, Garcia Espana F et al., Trazodone and valproate in patients discontinuing long-term benzodiazepine therapy: effects on

withdrawal symptoms and taper outcome, *Psychopharmacology (Berl)* (1999) 141: 1–5.

51. Rickels K, DeMartinis N, Garcia-Espana F et al., Imipramine and buspirone in treatment of patients with generalized anxiety disorder who are discontinuing long-term benzodiazepine therapy, *Am J Psychiatry* (2000) 157: 1973–9.

52. Zitman FG, Couvee JE, Chronic benzodiazepine use in general practice patients with depression: an evaluation of controlled treatment and taper-off: report on behalf of the Dutch Chronic Benzodiazepine Working Group, *Br J Psychiatry* (2001) 178: 317–24.

53. Spiegel DA, Bruce TJ, Gregg SF et al., Does cognitive behavior therapy assist slow-taper alprazolam discontinuation in panic disorder? *Am J Psychiatry* (1994) 151: 876–81.

54. Rickels K, Case WG, Schweizer EE et al., Low-dose dependence in chronic benzodiazepine users: a preliminary report on 119 patients, *Psychopharmacol Bull* (1986) 22: 407–15.

55. Griffiths RR, Lukas SE, Bradford LD et al., Self-injection of barbiturates and benzodiazepines in baboons, *Psychopharmacology (Berl)* (1981) 75: 101–9.

56. Bergman J, Johanson CE, The reinforcing properties of diazepam under several conditions in the rhesus monkey, *Psychopharmacology (Berl)* (1985) 86: 108–13.

57. Ator NA, Griffiths RR, Oral self-administration of triazolam, diazepam and ethanol in the baboon: drug reinforcement and benzodiazepine physical dependence, *Psychopharmacology (Berl)* (1992) 108: 301–12.

58. Ciraulo DA, Nace EP, Benzodiazepine treatment of anxiety or insomnia in substance abuse patients, *Am J Addict* (2000) 9: 276–9; discussion 80–4.

59. Cowley DS, Roy-Byrne PP, Godon C et al., Response to diazepam in sons of alcoholics, *Alcohol Clin Exp Res* (1992) 16: 1057–63.

60. de Wit H, Diazepam preference in males with and without an alcoholic first-degree relative, *Alcohol Clin Exp Res* (1991) 15: 593–600.

61. Caplan RD, Andrews FM, Conway TL et al., Social effects of diazepam use: a longitudinal field study, *Soc Sci Med* (1985) 21: 887–98.

62. Ciraulo DA, Barnhill JG, Ciraulo AM et al., Alterations in pharmacodynamics of anxiolytics in abstinent alcoholic men: subjective responses, abuse liability, and electroencephalographic effects of alprazolam, diazepam, and buspirone, *J Clin Pharmacol* (1997) 37: 64–73.

63. Abi-Dargham A, Krystal JH, Anjilvel S et al., Alterations of benzodiazepine receptors in type II alcoholic subjects measured with SPECT and [123I]iomazenil, *Am J Psychiatry* (1998) 155: 1550–5.

64. Behar KL, Rothman DL, Petersen KF et al., Preliminary evidence of low cortical GABA levels in localized 1H-MR spectra of alcohol-dependent and hepatic encephalopathy patients, *Am J Psychiatry* (1999) 156: 952–4.

65. Freund G, Ballinger WE, Jr., Decrease of benzodiazepine receptors in frontal cortex of alcoholics, *Alcohol* (1988) 5: 275–82.

66. Jaffe JH, Ciraulo DA, Nies A et al., Abuse potential of halazepam and of diazepam in patients recently treated for acute alcohol withdrawal, *Clin Pharmacol Ther* (1983) 34: 623–30.

67. Brown SS, Dundee JW, Clinical studies of induction agents. XXV. Diazepam, *Br J Anaesth* (1968) 40: 108–12.

68. Shader RI, Greenblatt DJ, Triazolam and anterograde amnesia: all is not well in the Z-zone, *J Clin Psychopharmacol* (1983) 3: 273.

69. Curran HV, Tranquillising memories: a review of the effects of benzodiazepines on human memory, *Biol Psychol* (1986) 23: 179–213.

70. Ghoneim MM, Mewaldt SP, Effects of diazepam and scopolamine on storage, retrieval and organizational processes in memory, *Psychopharmacologia* (1975) 44: 257–62.

71. Ghoneim MM, Mewaldt SP, Berie JL et al., Memory and performance effects of single and 3-week administration of diazepam, *Psychopharmacology (Berl)* (1981) 73: 147–51.

72. Morris HH, 3rd, Estes ML, Traveler's amnesia. Transient global amnesia secondary to triazolam, *JAMA* (1987) 258: 945–6.

73. Sandyk R, Transient global amnesia induced by lorazepam, *Clin Neuropharmacol* (1985) 8: 297–8.

74. File SE, Lister RG, Do lorazepam-induced deficits in learning result from impaired rehearsal, reduced motivation or increased sedation? *Br J Clin Pharmacol* (1982) 14: 545–50.

75. Hommer DW, Matsuo V, Wolkowitz O et al., Benzodiazepine sensitivity in normal human subjects, *Arch Gen Psychiatry* (1986) 43: 542–51.

76. Roy-Byrne PP, Uhde TW, Holcomb H et al., Effects of diazepam on cognitive processes in normal subjects, *Psychopharmacology (Berl)* (1987) 91: 30–3.

77. Pomara N, Stanley B, Block R et al., Increased sensitivity of the elderly to the central depressant effects of diazepam, *J Clin Psychiatry* (1985) **46**: 185–7.

78. Subhan Z, Hindmarch I, The effects of midazolam in conjunction with alcohol on iconic memory and free-recall, *Neuropsychobiology* (1983) **9**: 230–4.

79. Tariot PN, Weingartner H, A psychobiologic analysis of cognitive failures. Structure and mechanisms, *Arch Gen Psychiatry* (1986) **43**: 1183–8.

80. Rickels K, Lucki I, Schweizer E et al., Psychomotor performance of long-term benzodiazepine users before, during, and after benzodiazepine discontinuation, *J Clin Psychopharmacol* (1999) **19**: 107–13.

81. Gorenstein C, Bernik MA, Pompeia S, Differential acute psychomotor and cognitive effects of diazepam on long-term benzodiazepine users, *Int Clin Psychopharmacol* (1994) **9**: 145–53.

82. Gladsjo JA, Rapaport MH, McKinney R et al., Absence of neuropsychologic deficits in patients receiving long-term treatment with alprazolam-XR for panic disorder, *J Clin Psychopharmacol* (2001) **21**: 131–8.

83. Tata PR, Rollings J, Collins M et al., Lack of cognitive recovery following withdrawal from long-term benzodiazepine use, *Psychol Med* (1994) **24**: 203–13.

84. Kilic C, Curran HV, Noshirvani H et al., Long-term effects of alprazolam on memory: a 3.5 year follow-up of agoraphobia/panic patients, *Psychol Med* (1999) **29**: 225–31.

85. Lader MH, Ron M, Petursson H, Computed axial brain tomography in long-term benzodiazepine users, *Psychol Med* (1984) **14**: 203–6.

86. Schmauss C, Krieg JC, Enlargement of cerebrospinal fluid spaces in long-term benzodiazepine abusers, *Psychol Med* (1987) **17**: 869–73.

87. Busto UE, Bremner KE, Knight K et al., Long-term benzodiazepine therapy does not result in brain abnormalities, *J Clin Psychopharmacol* (2000) **20**: 2–6.

88. Wang PS, Bohn RL, Glynn RJ et al., Hazardous benzodiazepine regimens in the elderly: effects of half-life, dosage, and duration on risk of hip fracture, *Am J Psychiatry* (2001) **158**: 892–8.

89. Herings RM, Stricker BH, de Boer A et al., Benzodiazepines and the risk of falling leading to femur fractures. Dosage more important than elimination half-life, *Arch Intern Med* (1995) **155**: 1801–7.

90. Passaro A, Volpato S, Romagnoni F et al., Benzodiazepines with different half-life and falling in a hospitalized population: The GIFA study. Gruppo Italiano di Farmacovigilanza nell'Anziano, *J Clin Epidemiol* (2000) **53**: 1222–9.

91. Pierfitte C, Macouillard G, Thicoipe M et al., Benzodiazepines and hip fractures in elderly people: case-control study, *BMJ* (2001) **322**: 704–8.

92. Mendelson WB, The use of sedative/hypnotic medication and its correlation with falling down in the hospital, *Sleep* (1996) **19**: 698–701.

93. Thapa PB, Gideon P, Cost TW et al., Antidepressants and the risk of falls among nursing home residents, *N Engl J Med* (1998) **339**: 875–82.

94. Rothschild AJ, Shindul R, Viguera A et al., Comparison of the frequency of behavioral disinhibition on alprazolam, clonazepam, or no benzodiazepine in hospitalized psychiatric patients, *J Clin Psychopharmacol* (2000) **20**: 7–11.

10

Buspirone and Antihistamines in the Treatment of Generalized Anxiety Disorder

Sarosh Khalid-Khan, Moira Rynn and Karl Rickels

Introduction

This chapter focuses on the efficacy and safety of the azapirone buspirone and to a lesser extent on the antihistamine hydroxyzine for the treatment of generalized anxiety disorder (GAD). Buspirone is the only non-selective serotonergic medication presently approved for the treatment of GAD in many countries. Buspirone acts as a partial agonist at the $5\text{-}HT_{1A}$ serotonin receptor subtype and its primary mechanism of action is thus not serotonin reuptake inhibition.[1] Buspirone is the only $5\text{-}HT_{1A}$ partial agonist with a favorable adverse event profile and demonstrated anxiolytic efficacy. Of several sedating antihistamines, only hydroxyzine has been tested in anxious outpatients. It is not approved by the FDA for treatment of GAD but has a claim for 'symptomatic relief of anxiety symptoms'.

Buspirone

Mechanism of action/pharmacokinetic properties

$5\text{-}HT_{1A}$ drugs such as buspirone, gepirone and others appear to act as partial agonists at the post-synaptic $5\text{-}HT_{1A}$ population of serotonin receptors located at the hippocampus, but as full agonists at the presynaptic $5\text{-}HT_{1A}$ serotonergic autoreceptors, located in the dorsal raphe nucleus.[1,2,3] Binding to these receptors enables these drugs to influence the activity of serotonergic neurons through receptor down-regulation. In addition buspirone has a moderate affinity for presynaptic dopamine D_2 receptors. It is not known, however, whether this affinity for dopamine receptors contributes to the anxiolytic properties of buspirone.[4] Chronic administration of the azapirones, as with traditional antidepressants, causes a down-regulation of $5\text{-}HT_2$ receptors, possibly explaining their moderate antidepressant properties. Buspirone has a short elimination half-life of 2–3 hours with a weakly active metabolite 1-(2-pyrimidinyl)–piperazine (1-PP) that does not itself bind to 5-HT$_{1A}$ receptors and has alpha-2-adrenergic antagonistic properties. There is no interaction between the binding of benzodiazepines and buspirone.[5]

Buspirone is 100% absorbed after oral administration.[6] The oral bioavailability is approximately 5% after extensive first-pass metabolism, and a linear relationship between acute oral dose and area under the plasma concentration-time curve (AUC) was demonstrated. The first-pass metabolism of buspirone[7] is decreased by taking food with buspirone, but the clinical significance of these findings is not known. Buspirone is > 95% bound to plasma proteins, with about 70% of the bound fraction binding to albumin and 30% to alpha 1-acid glycoprotein.[8] Buspirone undergoes extensive metabolism so that less than 1% of an administered dose is excreted unchanged in the urine. There are 7 major and 5 minor metabolites that have been identified, and the major metabolic pathways are hydroxylation and dealkylation. The elimination half-life ($t_{\frac{1}{2}}$) of buspirone in healthy subjects ranges from 2 to 11 hours.

Lack of sedation and abuse liability

Buspirone has a low potential for sedation. When single or multiple doses of 5 mg buspirone were given, much less daytime sedation was seen with buspirone than with alprazolam 0.5 mg, diazepam 5 mg or lorazepam 1mg.[9] Comparing buspirone with diazepam, sedation in subjects with a single 10 mg dose of buspirone was less marked than with the same dose of diazepam.[10] Several psychomotor and cognitive studies with healthy subjects demonstrate that buspirone does not have the same impairing psychomotor effects as the benzodiazepines.[10,11] Driving skills, using a driving simulator, are not affected by buspirone.[12,13] In tests of memory function, assessed as immediate and delayed recall, buspirone appears to have minimal effects when compared to the benzodiazepines. For example, in anxious subjects Lucki et al.[14] confirmed that an acute dose of the benzodiazepine diazepam (5mg) but not buspirone (5mg) caused significant (p < .02) impairment of delayed recall when compared to placebo. Immediate recall was not affected by either medication.

Buspirone has no potential for abuse or dependence. For example, in individuals with a history of drug abuse, buspirone (15, 30, 60 and 120 mg/70kg) was rated by subjects as significantly 'less liked' than lorazepam (1, 2, 4 and 8 mg/70 kg).[15] In fact, the higher the dose of buspirone the more subjects reported 'disliking' the drug, whereas lorazepam produced a dose-dependent increase in drug 'liking'.

In contrast to the benzodiazepines, no discontinuation (withdrawal) symptoms have been demonstrated for buspirone. Rickels et al.[16] were the first group to search for possible evidence of physical dependence by treating chronically anxious patients for 6 months with either buspirone or the benzodiazepine clorazepate, substituting each drug with placebo abruptly at the end of treatment and maintaining patients on placebo for 4 weeks. Withdrawal symptoms were produced only by the benzodiazepine clorazepate and not by buspirone.

Adverse events

Newton et al.,[17] using data from 17 clinical trials, reported on frequency of adverse events for buspirone (n=477) and placebo (n=464). The most commonly reported adverse events were dizziness (12%), drowsiness (10%), nausea (8%), headache (6%), nervousness (5%), fatigue (4%), insomnia (3%), lightheadedness (3%), dry mouth (3%), and excitement (2%). However, patients receiving placebo also reported drowsiness, insomnia, fatigue and dry mouth at similar frequency. Adverse event reporting did not appear to be age-related. Sexual dysfunction was not reported with buspirone; in fact, improvement of sexual dysfunction caused by persistent anxiety,[18] or by selective serotonin reuptake inhibitors (SSRIs)[19] has been reported, perhaps related to the alpha-2 antagonistic effect of the metabolites. Other alpha-2 antagonists have been shown to promote sexual function.

There is very little published data on buspirone overdose, and the data that are available suggest that buspirone is not toxic in overdose. For example, in one study of 25 cases overdosing on buspirone, 10 subjects had taken buspirone alone. Drowsiness was the most commonly reported symptom. Forty-eight percent of patients had no symptoms, 40% had minor symptoms, 8% had moderate symptoms and 1 patient died. The patient who died was on a tricyclic antidepressant, which was the most likely cause of death. No deaths have been associated with an overdose of buspirone alone.[17]

In treatment-resistant depression, buspirone has been used to augment the antidepressant effect of SSRIs without any adverse effects.[20] Nevertheless, when combining serotonergic medications one must be careful to examine for the possibility of the development of a serotonergic syndrome. No interactions were observed in healthy subjects when buspirone was combined with benzodiazepines[21,22] or alcohol.[23] However, the addition of grapefruit juice,[24] significantly increased buspirone plasma concentrations, probably via inhibition of the cytochrome P-450, $3A_4$ iso-enzyme. While the use of benzodiazepines can be problematic in people with respiratory diseases because of the drugs' propensity to cause respiratory depression, buspirone does not cause respiratory depression.[25,26]

Therapeutic efficacy in generalized anxiety disorder

GAD is often a chronic condition, which interferes with the daily functioning of patients. It has a waxing and waning course interspersed with long intervals in which the patient is relatively free of anxiety. GAD has been treated with various psychotherapeutic approaches and medications. The acute phase of anxiety in chronically anxious patients is clearly managed best by anxiolytic medications like the benzodiazepines. However, it is very difficult for most chronically anxious patients to sustain remission of their anxiety symptoms. Less than 50% of chronically anxious patients will have sustained remission of symptoms after stopping acute medication treatment.[27] Some chronically anxious patients may need to be treated for years. Benzodiazepines have been used for a long time for the treatment of anxiety; however, they are sedating and with prolonged use can cause physical dependence.[28] Consequently, the pharmaceutical industry has searched for non-benzodiazepine anxiolytics, a search that eventually produced buspirone.

In the past 20 years a number of double-blind studies, some of them placebo-controlled, have confirmed buspirone's efficacy in the alleviation of anxiety symptoms in patients suffering from GAD. Most of these were placebo lead-in, randomized, double-blind studies designed to minimize any placebo effect. The primary measure of efficacy was the Hamilton Anxiety Rating Scale (HAM-A).[29] Patients were generally required to have a HAM-A score of at least 18 when admitted to the trial. Some of the studies were supported by competitors of the manufacturer of buspirone using buspirone as an active control in the evaluation of new anxiolytics.[30,31] The results observed by Pollack et al.[30]

in a large multi-site trial with HAM-A as the primary efficacy variable are given for 3- and 6-week endpoints in Figure 10.1. These data support earlier studies that buspirone's onset of action is rather gradual.[16,31,32,33]

All published placebo-controlled, double-blind trials, usually of 4–6 week duration, that also included a benzodiazepine showed that buspirone had equal efficacy to a standard benzodiazepine and significantly better response than placebo.[29,32,33,34,35,36,37,38,39] Additional non-placebo-controlled, double-blind studies compared buspirone against several benzodiazepines and also demonstrated equal efficacy for both treatments.[33,40,41,42,43,44] The majority of buspirone GAD studies used DSM III and not the more stringent DSM-IV

criteria. One of the most salient clinical features of buspirone, compared with the benzodiazepines, is its *gradual, relatively slow onset of action*, with many patients taking 4–6 weeks to respond.[16,30,31,32,38] This slow onset of action makes buspirone less useful for the treatment of transient, situational, or acute anxiety and may account for the perception by some clinicians that buspirone is a slightly less effective anxiolytic than the benzodiazepines.[45] A similar slow onset of action has been reported for the treatment of anxiety symptoms with anti-depressants.[46,47] Buspirone's slow onset of action appears to be derived from its lack of sedative and muscle-relaxing properties, as well as its lack of action at the GABA receptor complex. Psychic symptoms of anxiety such as worry, anger, irritability, and difficulty concentrating, which are diagnostically considered core features of GAD in DSM-IV, respond faster to buspirone when compared to the benzodiazepines, while the reverse is true for somatic symptoms such as muscle tension and insomia.[35,38] Similar observations were made for antidepressants prescribed as anxiolytics.[31,46,47]

The observation that patients with GAD who also had sub-syndromal *depressive symptoms* frequently also improved in their depressive symptomatology during treatment with buspirone,[48] led to several studies being carried out with anxious, major depressed patients, using slightly higher daily doses than were used in GAD. All studies showed significantly more antidepressant efficacy for buspirone than for placebo.[49,50,51] Robinson et al.[52] combined these studies and confirmed marked improvement in depressive symptoms (Figure 10.2).

It must be stressed, however, that buspirone is not approved for the treatment of major depression and that its antidepressant effects were observed in anxious depressed patients only.

While most anxiolytic studies were conducted with patients ≤ 65 years of age, in a

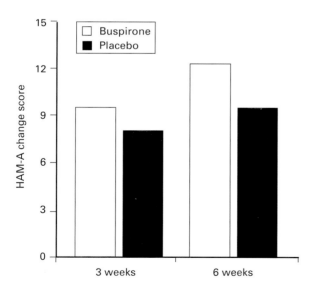

Figure 10.1 Clinical improvement: Hamilton Anxiety Scale change scores between baseline and 3 and 6 weeks of treatment; LOCF data set. Buspirone (n=108), placebo (n=110) comparison: 3 weeks p < .113; 6 weeks p < .043, two tailed. Data from Pollack et al.[30]

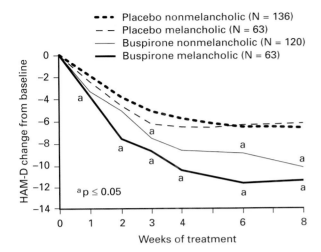

Figure 10.2 Effect of buspirone and placebo on 25-item Hamilton Depression Scale scores in major depression with anxiety. [a]p < 0.05; improvement significantly greater with buspirone. Data from Robinson et al.[52]

number of studies this age limitation did not exist and thus a large number of patients over age 65 were available for a comparison with patients under 65. These comparisons indicated that elderly patients respond similarly to buspirone as younger patients.[53,54,55] Much less is known about buspirone's usefulness in children. Only two open studies report on the use of buspirone in children and adolescents, and 'some' beneficial effects after 6 weeks of treatment[56,57] were observed.

Since buspirone does not exhibit cross-tolerance to the benzodiazepines, and thus does not block benzodiazepine withdrawal symptoms, patients should never be abruptly *switched from a benzodiazepine to buspirone*. When switching benzodiazepine-treated patients to buspirone, it is beneficial to initiate buspirone therapy concurrently for 2–4 weeks before tapering off the benzodiazepine gradually. Some studies, in which the benzodiazepine was abruptly replaced with buspirone, have shown no

benefit for buspirone facilitating benzodiazepine withdrawal,[58] while other studies have shown some beneficial results when buspirone was started several weeks before the benzodiazepine taper process was initiated.[59,60,61]

Schweizer et al.[62] were the first authors to observe that *prior benzodiazepine use* affected treatment outcome in that patients treated with buspirone who had received prior benzodiazepines responded less well than those previously untreated with a benzodiazepine. At that time the authors speculated that this effect may have been related to the treatment expectations of patients based on earlier experience with benzodiazepines, which may have prejudiced clinical outcome. Particularly, benzodiazepine-treated patients may have expected sedation and/or euphoria side effects they hardly experienced with buspirone. More recently, DeMartinis et al.[63] reviewed a large data set and examined the response to buspirone treatment as a function of patients who were never treated with benzodiazepines, were remotely treated (> 1 month ago), or were recently treated with benzodiazepines (< 1 month ago). Results clearly indicated that treatment response to buspirone was only impaired in patients who had recently (< 1 month) terminated benzodiazepine treatment but not in patients who had either never been treated or had been treated several months ago with a benzodiazepine (Figure 10.3). Therefore, the recommendation can be made that initiation of buspirone therapy in patients recently on benzodiazepines should be undertaken cautiously and be combined with appropriate patient education.

Dosage and administration

The recommended initial dosage of buspirone is 15 mg/day administered in 2–3 divided

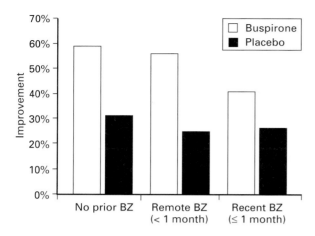

Figure 10.3 Clinical global improvement (moderate/marked) with buspirone after 4 weeks of treatment (LOCF data set) as a function of prior benzodiazepine use. BU = Buspirone (n=252); PL = placebo (n=235). Buspirone/placebo differences, based on chi square, two tailed: no prior BZ p< 0.001; remote (> 4 weeks) prior BZ p < 0.005; recent (< 4 weeks) prior BZ p < 0.065 Data from DeMartinis et al.[63]

doses. The dosage should be increased to 30 mg daily to achieve an optimal therapeutic response. The recommended maximum daily dosage is 45 mg in the UK and 60 mg in the US.

There are no firm recommendations regarding dosage adjustments in patients with hepatic or renal insufficiency. Although there appears to be some reduction in the elimination of buspirone or the active N-dealkylated metabolite (1-PP) in such patients, inter-patient variation in pharmacokinetic parameters is substantial. Nevertheless, dosage adjustments may be necessary in patients with severe renal or hepatic impairment. No age-related dosage adjustments are necessary in elderly patients.

Conclusion

A large amount of pre-clinical and clinical data is available in the literature, demonstrating buspirone's safety and efficacy in the treatment of GAD patients. It is the first non-benzodiazepine anxiolytic introduced into psychiatry. It causes little sedation and consequently has no negative effects on psychomotor and cognitive functions, including memory and driving skills. It is well tolerated and safe in overdose. Patients do not suffer discontinuation or withdrawal symptoms

Table 10.1
Clinical properties of buspirone
• Efficacy in GAD similar to the benzodiazepines
• Minimal sedation
• No abuse or dependency problem with long-term use, no euphoria
• Few adverse events, well tolerated in overdose, and no interaction with alcohol
• Preliminary evidence that buspirone may help and not hinder acquiring new coping skills
• Slow, gradual onset of efficacy: therefore, not indicated for the acute treatment of transient or situational anxiety, but well indicated for the long-term ($\geq$ 4 weeks) treatment of GAD patients
• Psychic symptoms improve earlier than somatic symptoms
• Effective in treating anxiety with co-existing depressive symptoms
• Switching from benzodiazepines to buspirone should be done cautiously. Start buspirone therapy for 2–4 weeks prior to benzodiazepine taper initiation.

when buspirone is abruptly stopped, even after many months of treatment. Reassessment of continued need for buspirone therapy is therefore simple without the risk of rebound anxiety, a phenomenon that frequently makes temporary discontinuation of benzodiazepines a challenge. Since buspirone does not interact with alcohol, it is a safe alternative to the benzodiazepines for those anxious patients who request to be able to have an occasional alcohol intake.

Controlled clinical trials have demonstrated buspirone's anxiolytic efficacy to be equal to that of the benzodiazepines and significantly better than that of placebo. The perception among some clinicians that buspirone has slightly lower anxiolytic efficacy than the benzodiazepines may well be related to its relatively slow onset of action and its lack of sedative effects, effects that might be particularly missed by patients recently treated with a benzodiazepine. Consequently, patients switched from a benzodiazepine to buspirone should be well prepared and informed about what to expect from buspirone therapy and how buspirone differs from the benzodiazepines. Patients should be informed that buspirone is less sedating and has a more gradual onset of action than the benzodiazepines. Patients should be encouraged to give buspirone some time to work. Patients can be further assured that if they are in need of prolonged therapy, buspirone does not cause physical dependence and withdrawal symptoms upon discontinuation, and thus is a safer drug than the benzodiazepines for long-term treatment.[16] Finally, patients may be informed that there is preliminary evidence that long-term treatment with buspirone, in contrast to long-term treatment with benzodiazepines, does not decrease the ability to learn new coping skills.[27,64]

Many clinicians prefer buspirone to the benzodiazepines for the long-term (more than 4 weeks) treatment of anxious patients for two main reasons. One reason is the low level of adverse events, the lack of sedation and the lack of withdrawal symptoms on abrupt treatment discontinuation, and the other reason is buspirone's moderate antidepressant properties which allow treatment of the many anxious patients who also suffer from secondary depressive symptoms at a diagnostic subthreshold level. Since buspirone does not have the fast onset of action of the benzodiazepines, it is not indicated for the short-term (i.e. 1 to 14 days) treatment of situational or temporary anxiety conditions. Many clinicians use a gradual dose titration of buspirone, starting with 10 mg/day and increasing weekly by 10 mg increments up to 40–60 mg prescribed b.i.d. or t.i.d. This regime produces few unwanted side effects.

Hydroxyzine

Sedating antihistamines such as diphenhydramine have been used for many years as over-the-counter (OTC) sleep-aids.[65,66] Several combinations of scopolamine and antihistamines were also promoted in the US prior to 1975 as OTC 'tranquilizers' and 'sedatives' before being forced off the market by the FDA for lack of proven efficacy. Rickels and Hesbacher conducted the only placebo-controlled, double-blind trial using Compoz, a combinative of scopolamine and the antihistamines methapyrilene and pyrilamine, representative of many OTC 'tranquilizers', and found Compoz devoid of any anti-anxiety properties.[67]

The antihistamine hydroxyzine is the only antihistamine that was studied in the early

1960s as an anxiolytic, and in the US has an indication for use in the symptomatic relief of 'anxiety symptoms and tensions associated with psycho-neurotic condition or physical disease state'. Hydroxyzine acts as an antagonist at H_1 receptors and to a lesser extent at muscarinic receptors and 5-HT$_2$ receptors. It has even less binding to alpha-1 and dopamine-2 receptors.[68,69] Clinical trials conducted in the late 1960s and early 1970s demonstrated some anti-anxiety and anti-tension effects for hydroxyzine, but only when prescribed at rather high daily dosages of 300–400 mg/day. These studies are summarized by Barranco and Bridger.[70] Many of these early trials suffered, as most trials of that time, from lack of rigid methodology and diagnostic precision, and small sample sizes. The duration of all studies was 4 weeks or less.

Three placebo-controlled trials in a daily dosage range of 300–400 mg of hydroxyzine, given in divided doses, were conducted at that time, one by Breslow[71] in anxious prison inmates, one by Goldberg & Finnerty[72] in anxious family practice patients, and one large study by Rickels et al.[73] in anxious out-patients. The study by Rickels et al. also included the benzodiazepine chlordiazepoxide as a control agent. Both hydroxyzine (400 mg/day) and chlordiazepoxide (40 mg/day) caused significantly more improvement than placebo after 4 weeks of treatment (p< .05). Hydroxyzine, however, produced more side effects (primarily sedation, and such autonomic symptoms as dizziness and dry mouth). When patients were asked to state whether they preferred the study drug to their previous drug, 71% of patients preferred the chlordiazepoxide, 60% hydroxyzine and 37% placebo (p < .05). Today hydroxyzine is used for the treatment of such allergic reactions as urticaria and pruritis. It may produce central nervous system (CNS) depression when added

to alcohol, narcotics, analgesics, and CNS depressants.

A hiatus of over 20 years occurred in which no further studies were conducted with hydroxyzine in psychiatry. In the early 1990s interest was again generated in hydroxyzine by a large multi-site family practice study conducted in France, and published in 1995.[74] This study used a sample size of 110 and compared a low dose of hydroxyzine (50 mg/day), given in divided doses, to placebo. Patients were diagnosed as suffering from GAD according to DSM-III-R criteria and had to have a Hamilton Anxiety Scale (HAM-A) score at intake of 20. Statistically significant differences in favor of hydroxyzine were present at week 4 but not at week 1, and this improvement was maintained for 1 additional week while patients received a placebo. Thus, no evidence for discontinuation symptoms or withdrawal symptoms was observed after 4 weeks of hydroxyzine treatment. The Hamilton Anxiety Scale change score at week 4 was 11.5 for the hydroxyzine group and 6.6 for the placebo group (p< .01).

This French multicentre family practice trial was followed by a second family practice multicentre trial (n=243), now also involving a few practice sites from the United Kingdom (48 French and 14 English family practice sites).[75] Buspirone 20 mg/day was used as an active control. Study duration was again 4 weeks and the dosage of hydroxyzine was again 50 mg/day. At week 4 hydroxyzine differed significantly from placebo (p < .01) on the Hamilton Anxiety Scale total score but buspirone did not. Four-week HAM-A change scores were 11.8 for hydroxyzine, 8.8 for buspirone and 7.2 for placebo. Interestingly, in all secondary assessment measures such as the Hospital Anxiety and Depression Scale (HAD), the Montgomery Asberg Rating Scale (MADRS) and the Ferrari Anxiety Scale, not only hydroxyzine but also buspirone differed significantly from placebo. For example, the MADRS change score was 6.6 for hydroxyzine, 6.5 for buspirone and 3.9 for placebo (p< .001). Since buspirone has a gradual onset of anxiolytic action, it should not be surprising that at 4 weeks its anxiolytic efficacy was not yet fully demonstrated. No data are available in the literature on the efficacy and safety of hydroxyzine when prescribed for periods over 4 weeks, including whether or not discontinuation symptoms occur.

Conclusion

In summary, for patients needing anxiolytic treatment and who are adverse to using benzodiazepines even for the short term (< 4 weeks), use of hydroxyzine might possibly represent a potential alternative to the benzodiazepines in the treatment of generalized anxiety symptoms, particularly if physicians are concerned about alcohol intake and chronic use. Before this conclusion can be drawn, however, an explanation must be provided of why in the earlier trials in the late 1960s and early 1970s dosages under 200 mg/day were found ineffective as anxiolytics while in the two most recent studies, the very low daily dose of only 50 mg was found effective. Earlier studies clearly lacked diagnostic precision and may have included many rather acutely anxious patients who today would be diagnosed as having adjustment disorders or acute stress reactions. Clearly only controlled research, conducted with well-diagnosed GAD patients, using a longer than 4-week duration of treatment and comparing several dosages of hydroxyzine with placebo and with a standard anxiolytic agent could provide answers to this important clinical question. Therefore, recommendations for the use of hydroxyzine must await the results of such studies.

References

1. Eison MS, Azapirones: mechanism of action in anxiety and depression, *Drug Ther* (1990) **20** (Suppl):3–8

2. De Montigny C, Blier P, Potentiation of 5-HT neurotransmission by short-term lithium: in vivo electrophysiological studies, *Clin Neuropharmacol* (1992) 15:610A–611A

3. Eison AS, Temple DL, Buspirone: Review of its pharmacology and current perspectives on its mechanism of action, *Am J Med* (1986) **80**:1–9

4. Pecknold JC, Serotonin 5-HT1A agonists: a comparative review, *CNS Drugs* (1994) 234–51

5. Goa KL, Ward A, Buspirone: A preliminary review of its pharmacological properties and therapeutic efficacy as an anxiolytic, *Drugs* (1986) 32:114–29

6. Jajoo HK, Mayol RF, LaBudde JA, et al, Metabolism of the antianxiety drug buspirone in human subjects, *Drug Metab Dispos* (1989) 17:634–40

7. Mayol RF, Gammans RE, Mackenthun AV, et al, The effect of food on the bioavailability of buspirone HCI [abstract], *Clin Res* (1983) 31:631a

8. Gammans RE, Mayol RF, Labudde JA, Metabolism and disposition of buspirone. *Am J Med* (1986) **80** (Suppl 3B):41–51

9. Dement WC, Seidel WF, Cohen SA, et al, Effects of alprazolam, buspirone and diazepam on daytime sedation and performance, *Drug Invest* (1991) 3:148–56

10. Boulenger JP, Squillace K, Simon P, et al, Buspirone and diazepam: comparison of subjective, psychomotor and biological effects, *Neuropsychobiology* (1989) 22:83–9

11. Schaffler K, Klausnitzer W, Placebo-controlled study on acute and subchronic effects of buspirone versus bromazepam utilizing psychomotor and cognitive assessments in healthy volunteers, *Pharmacopsychiatry* (1989) 22:26–33

12. Moskowitz H, Smiley A, Effects of chronically administered buspirone and diazepam on driving-related skills performance, *J Clin Psychiatry* (1982) 43:45–55

13. van Laar MW, Volkerts ER, van Willigenburg AP, Therapeutic effects and effects on actual driving performance of chronically administered buspirone and diazepam in anxious outpatients, *J Clin Psychopharmacol* (1992) 12:86–95

14. Lucki I, Rickels K, Giesecke A, Geller A, Differential effects of the anxiolytic drugs, diazepam and buspirone on memory function, *Br J Clin Pharmac* (1987) 23:207–11

15. Sellers EM, Schneiderman JF, Romacch MK, et al, Comparative drug effects and abuse liability of lorazepam, buspirone, and secobarbital in nondependent subjects, *J Clin Psychopharmacol* (1992) 12:79–85

16. Rickels K, Schweizer E, Csanalosi I, Case WG, Chung H, Long-term treatment of anxiety and risk of withdrawal: prospective comparison of clorazepate and buspirone, *Arch Gen Psychiatry* (1988) 45:444–50

17. Newton RE, Marunycz JD, Alderdice MT, et al, Review of the side-effect profile of buspirone, *Am J Med* (1986) 80 (Suppl 3B):17–21

18. Othmer E, Othmer SC, Effect of buspirone on sexual dysfunction in patients with generalized anxiety disorder, *J Clin Psychiatry* (1987) 48:201–3

19. Norden MJ, Buspirone treatment of sexual dysfunction associated with selective serotonin re-uptake inhibitors, *Depression* (1994) 2:109–12

20. Jacobsen FM, Possible augmentation of antidepressant response by buspirone, *J Clin Psychiatry* (1991) 52:217–20

21. Boulenger J-P, Gram LF, Jolicoeur FB, et al, Repeated administration of buspirone: absence of pharmacodynamic or pharmacokinetic interaction with triazolam, *Human Psychopharmacology* (1993) 8:117–24

22. Buch AB, Van Harken DR, Seidehamel RJ, et al, A study of pharmacokinetic interaction between buspirone and alprazolam at steady state, *J Clin Pharmacol* (1993) 33:1104–9

23. Erwin CW, Linnoila M, Hartwell J, et al, Effects of buspirone and diazepam, alone and in combination with alcohol, on skilled performance and evoked potentials, *J Clin Psychopharmacol* (1986) 6:199–209

24. Lilja JJ, Kivisto KT, Backman JT, Lamberg TS, Neuvonen PJ, Grapefruit juice substantially increases plasma concentrations of buspirone, *Clin Pharmacol Ther* (1998) 64:655-60

25. Craven J, Sutherland A, Buspirone for anxiety disorders in patients with severe lung disease [letter], *Lancet* (1991) 338:249

26. Rapaport DM, Greenberg HE, Goldring RM, Differing effects of the anxiolytic agents buspirone and diazepam on control of breathing, *Clin Pharmacol Ther* (1991) 49:394–401

27. Rickels K, Schweizer E, The clinical course and long-term management of generalized anxiety disorder, *J Clin Psychopharmacol* (1990) 10:101S–110S

28. American Psychiatric Association. Benzodiazepine Dependence, Toxicity, and Abuse: A Task Force Report of the American Psychiatric Association (Washington, DC, APA, 1990)

29. Hamilton MA, The assessment of anxiety states by rating, *Br J Med Psychol* (1959) 32:50–5

30. Pollack MH, Worthington JJ, Manfro GG, Otto MW, Zucker BG, Abecarnil for the treatment of generalized anxiety disorder: A placebo-controlled comparison of two dosage ranges of abecarnil and buspirone, *J Clin Psychiatry* (1997) 58(11):19–23

31. Davidson JR, Dupont RL, Hedges D, Haskins JT, Efficacy, safety, and tolerability of venlafaxine extended release and buspirone in outpatients with generalized anxiety disorder, *J Clin Psychiatry* (1999) 60:528–35

32. Enkelmann R, Alprazolam vs buspirone in the treatment of outpatients with generalized anxiety disorder, *Psychopharmacology* (1991) 105:428–32

33. Murphy SM, Owen R, Tyrer P, Comparative assessment of efficacy and withdrawal symptoms after 6 and 12 weeks' treatment with diazepam or buspirone, *Br J Psychiatry* (1989) 154:529–34

34. Goldberg HL, Finnerty RJ, The comparative efficacy of buspirone and diazepam in the treatment of anxiety, *Am J Psychiatry* (1979) 136:1184–7

35. Rickels K, Wiseman K, Norstad N et al, Buspirone and diazepam in anxiety: a controlled study, *J Clin Psychiatry* (1982) 43:81–6

36. Boehm C, Placchi M, Stallone F, Gammans RE, Alms DR, Shrotriya RC, Robinson RS, A double-blind comparison of buspirone, clobazepam, and placebo in patients with anxiety treated in a general practice setting, *J Clin Psychopharmacol* (1990) 10:385–425

37. Laakman G, Schule C, Lorkowski G, Baghai T, Kuhn K, Ehrentraut S, Buspirone and lorazepam in the treatment of generalized anxiety disorder in outpatients, *Psychopharmacology* (1998) 136: 357–66

38. Pecknold JC, Matas M, Howarth BG et al, Evaluation of buspirone as an antianxiety agent: buspirone and diazepam vs placebo, *Am J Psychiatry* (1989) 34:766–71

39. Cohn JB, Rickels K, A pooled, double-blind comparison of the effects of buspirone, diazepam and placebo in women with chronic anxiety, *Curr Med Res Opin* (1989) 11:304–20

40. Sacchetti E, Zerbini O, Banfi F et al, Overlap of buspirone with lorazepam, diazepam and bromazepam in patients with generalized anxiety disorder: findings from a controlled, multicenter, double-blind study, *Human Psychopharmacol* (1994) 9:409–22

41. Dimitriou EC, Parashos AJ, Giouzepas JS, Buspirone versus alprazolam: a double-blind comparative study of their efficacy, adverse effects and withdrawal symptoms, *Drug Invest* (1992) 4:316–21

42. Strand M, Hetta J, Rosen A et al, A double-blind, controlled trial in primary care patients with generalized anxiety: a comparison between buspirone and oxazepam, *J Clin Psychiatry* (1990) 51 (Suppl):40–5

43. Wheatley D, Buspirone, Multicenter efficacy study, *J Clin Psychiatry* (1982) 43:92–4

44. Cohn JB, Bowden CL, Fisher JG, Rodos J, Double-blind comparison of buspirone and clorazepate in anxious outpatients, *Am J Med* (1986) 80:10–16

45. Deakin JFW, A review of the clinical efficacy of 5-HT$_{1A}$ agonists in anxiety and depression, *J Psychopharmacol* (1993) 7:283–9

46. Rickels K, Downing R, Schweizer E, Hassman H, Antidepressants for the treatment of generalized anxiety disorder: A placebo-controlled comparison of imipramine, trazodone, and diazepam, *Arch Gen Psychiatry* (1993) 50:884–95

47. Rickels K, Pollack MH, Sheehan DV, Haskins JT, Efficacy of extended-release venlafaxine in nondepressed outpatients with generalized anxiety disorder, *Am J Psychiatry* (2000) 157:968–74

48. Feighner JP, Merideth CH, Hendrickson GA, A double-blind comparison of buspirone and diazepam in outpatients with generalized anxiety disorder, *J Clin Psychiatry* (1982) 43:103–7

49. Rickels K, Amsterdam JD, Clary C, Puzzuoli G, Schweizer E, Buspirone in major depression: a controlled study, *J Clin Psychiatry* (1991) 52:34–8

50. Fabre LF, Buspirone in the management of major depression: a placebo-controlled comparison, *J Clin Psychiatry* (1990) 51 (Suppl):55-61

51. Sramek JJ, Tansman M, Suri A et al, Efficacy of buspirone in generalized anxiety disorder with coexisting mild depressive symptoms, *J Clin Psychiatry* (1996) 57:287–91

52. Robinson DS, Rickels K, Feighner J, Fabre LF, Gammans RE, Shrotriya RC, Alms CR, Andray JJ, Messina ME, Clinical effects of the 5-HT$_{1A}$ partial agonists in depression: a composite analysis of buspirone in the treatment of depressions, *J Clin Psychopharmacol* (1990) 10:67S–76S

53. Goldberg RJ, The use of buspirone in geriatric patients, *J Clin Psychiatry* (1994) 12:31–2

54. Boehm C, Robinson DS, Gammans RE et al, Buspirone therapy in anxious elderly patients: a controlled clinical trial, *J Clin Psychopharmacol* (1990) 10(Suppl):47–51

55. Robinson D, Napoliello MJ, Schenk J, The safety and usefulness of buspirone as an anxiolytic drug in the elderly versus young patients, *Clin Therap* (1988) 10:740–6

56. Kutcher SP, Reiter S, Gardener DM et al, The pharmacotherapy of anxiety disorders in children and adolescents, *Psychiatr Clin North Am* (1992) 15:41–66

57. Simeon JG, Knott VJ, Dubois C et al, Buspirone therapy of mixed anxiety disorders in childhood and adolescence: A pilot study, *J Child Adolesc Psychopharmacol* (1994) 4:159–70

58. Schweizer E, Rickels K, Failure of buspirone to manage benzodiazepine withdrawal, *Am J Psychiatry* (1986) 143:1590–2

59. Udelman HD, Udelman DL, Concurrent use of buspirone in anxious patients during withdrawal from alprazolam therapy, *J Clin Psychiatry* (1990) 51:9(Suppl):46–50

60. Chiaie R, Pancheri P, Cassacchia M et al, Assessment of the efficacy of buspirone in patients affected by generalized anxiety disorder, shifting to buspirone from prior treatment with lorazepam: a placebo-controlled, double-blind study, *J Clin Psychopharmacology* (1995) 15:12–19

61. Rickels K, DeMartinis N, Garcia-Espana F, Greenblat D, Mandos L, Rynn M, Imipramine and buspirone in treatment of patients with generalized anxiety disorder who are discontinuing long-term

benzodiazepine therapy, *Am J Psychiatry* (2000) 157:1973–9

62. Schweizer E, Rickels K, Lucki I, Resistance to the anti-anxiety effect of buspirone in patients with a history of benzodiazepine use, *N Engl J Med* (1986) 314:719–20

63. DeMartinis N, Rynn M, Rickels K, Mandos L, Prior benzodiazepine use and buspirone response in the treatment of generalized anxiety disorder, *J Clin Psychiatry* (2000) 61:91–4

64. Scheibe G, Four-year follow-up in 40 outpatients with anxiety disorder: buspirone versus lorazepam, *Eur J Psychiat* (1996) 10:25-34

65. Department of Health, Education and Welfare, Food and Drug Administration, Over-the-counter night-time sleep-aid and stimulant products. Tentative final orders. Federal register. (1978) 42:25544

66. Rickels K, Morris RJ, Newman H, Rosenfeld H, Schiller H, Weinstock R, Diphenhydramine in insomniac family practice patients: A double-blind study, *J Clin Pharmacol* (1983) 23:235-42

67. Rickels K, Hesbacher PT, Over-the-Counter Daytime Sedatives. A controlled study, *JAMA* (1973) 223:29–33

68. Kubo N, Shirakawa T, Kuno T, Tanaka C, Antimuscarinic effects of antihistamines: quantitative evaluation by receptor-binding assay, *Jpn J Pharmacol* (1987) 43:277–81

69. Snyder SH, Snowman AM, Receptor effects of cetirizine, *Ann Allergy* (1987) 59:4–8

70. Barranco SF, Bridger W, Treatment of anxiety with oral hydroxyzine: An overview, *Current Therapeutic Research* (1977) 22:217–27

71. Breslow IH, Evaluation of hydroxyzine pamoate concentrate as an ataractic: double-blind cross-over study in a neurotic male prison group, *Curr Ther Res* (1968) 10:421–7

72. Goldberg L, Finnerty RJ, The use of hydroxyzine in the treatment of anxiety neurosis, *Psychosomatics* (1973) 14:38–41

73. Rickels K, Gordon PE, Zamostein BB, Case W, Hutchinson J, Chung H, Hydroxyzine and chlordiaxepoxide in anxious neurotic outpatients – a collaborative controlled study, *Compr Psychiatry* (1970) 11:457–74

74. Darcis T, Ferreri M, Natens J, Burtin B, Deram P and the French GP Study Group for Hydroxyzine, A multicentre double-blind, placebo-controlled study investigating the anxiolytic efficacy of hydroxyzine in patients with generalized anxiety, *Hum Psychopharmacol* (1995) 10:181–7

75. Lader M, Scotto JC, A multicentre double-blind comparison of hydroxyzine, buspirone and placebo in patients with generalized anxiety disorder, *Psychopharmacology* (1998) 139:402–6

11

Antidepressants in the Treatment of Generalized Anxiety Disorder

Ashok Raj and David V Sheehan

Background

Generalized anxiety disorder (GAD) was born in 1980, in part out of a misunderstanding of treatment effects. It was delivered by a committee and has since metamorphosed into a disorder with a new configuration. The DSM III committee carved the older diagnostic category anxiety neurosis into two principal disorders, panic disorder and GAD.[1] The rationale for this split was the observation that the tricyclic antidepressant, imipramine, was effective against spontaneous panic attacks while benzodiazepines were not believed to be effective in this disorder. They created GAD as a residual disorder to accommodate patients who did not have spontaneous panic attacks, but who were generally anxious. Using a model of 'pharmacological dissection', panic disorder was created as the tricyclic sensitive 'antidepressant', but benzodiazepine non-responsive disorder, while GAD was created as the benzodiazepine sensitive but tricyclic non-responsive disorder. Historically, benzodiazepines have been the mainstay of treatment for GAD.[2-6]

The clinical trial evidence in support of this split was weak. The best evidence supported the view that tricyclics were effective in spontaneous panic attacks.[7] The evidence suggesting tricyclics or other antidepressants were not effective in GAD and that benzodiazepines were not effective in panic disorder was not strong at the time.

In 1982,[8] 1984[9] and 1984,[10] Sheehan demonstrated that the benzodiazepine alprazolam was effective in panic disorder. Chouinard et al also made this observation in 1982.[11] Ballenger et al in 1988 and Katschnig et al in 1995 replicated these results.[12,13] In 1983, Rickels et al demonstrated that the benzodiazepine alprazolam was effective in GAD.[14] In 1989, Sheehan et al, in two parallel and concurrent studies by the same research team, demonstrated that the triazolo-benzodiazepine adinazolam (very similar to alprazolam) was effective in both panic disorder and GAD.[15,16]. However, the dose of adinazolam needed to treat GAD effectively (95.8±28mg) was higher than the dose needed to treat panic disorder (91.8±28.4 mg).[15,16] In spite of this, the adinazolam delivered lower (better) endpoint scores on the Hamilton Anxiety Scale in panic disorder (6.8±7) than the endpoint Hamilton Anxiety Scale (HAM-A) scores in GAD (9.3±5.8).[15,16] This suggested that contrary to prior assumptions and the prevailing opinion of many, a benzodiazepine (adinazolam) was less effective in GAD than in panic disorder and required higher doses in GAD than in panic disorder. The observation that adinazolam doses were higher in GAD than in panic disorder is contrary to all other data reported in the literature. In 1986, the FDA approved buspirone, a partial agonist of $5HT_{1A}$ receptors, for the treatment of 'anxiety' with a symptom cluster similar to GAD. However, experienced clinicians considered it weak and not reliably effective. Since then the FDA has not approved any other $5HT_{1A}$ agonist in any anxiety disorder – a testimony to the relative weakness of the class.

Turning point in treatment

The turning point in the treatment of GAD came with a double blind placebo-controlled study in 1993 by Rickels et al[17] comparing two antidepressants (the tricyclic imipramine and trazodone) with diazepam. They found that the tricyclic antidepressant imipramine was significantly better than placebo in the treatment of 230 non-depressed GAD patients over 8 weeks. In addition, imipramine showed a trend to be significantly better on the primary outcome measure (HAM-A) scale and was statistically superior to the benzodiazepine on the psychic anxiety factor of the HAM-A.[17] Psychic anxiety includes the items of worry, anxious mood, tension, irritability and concentration problems.[17]

Rickels et al also found that the benzo-diazepine diazepam and the tricyclic anti-depressant imipramine had identical endpoint HAM-A somatic anxiety factor scores, suggesting that they are equally effective against the somatic anxiety symptoms in GAD.[17] Thus, their data do not support the conclusion that benzodiazepines, after 8 weeks of treatment, are more effective against somatic anxiety than imipramine. In contrast, they found that diazepam does not lower the psychic anxiety factor score of the HAM-A significantly more than placebo, while imipramine does.[17] This suggests that the antidepressant imipramine is exerting its main effect in GAD against the psychic anxiety symptoms (worry, anxious mood, tension, concentration problems and irritability) and is a better anti-worry medication than the benzodiazepine. Patients treated with diazepam had an earlier response than those on imipramine, while those treated with both the antidepressants took longer to respond.[17] The mean maximum daily dose was 143 mg for imipramine, 255 mg for trazodone, and 26 mg for diazepam.[17]

These findings had important implications in the new DSM IV formulation of GAD.[18] They provided the first solid demonstration that, contrary to earlier opinion, the antidepressant imipramine was a better treatment for GAD than the anxiolytic benzodiazepine diazepam. DSM IV (1994) reformulated GAD as a syndrome with uncontrollable worry and anxiety about a variety of life events as its central focus, while reducing the number and importance of somatic and autonomic symptoms.[18]

The findings of Rickels et al in 1993 came at a time when a series of SSRIs and SNRIs were entering the market.[17] Recognition that antidepressants were better treatments for GAD than pure anxiolytics like benzodiazepines suggested that they might serve as better treatments for GAD than the older anxiolytics.

These findings by Sheehan et al[8–10] and Rickels et al[17] called into question prior assumptions about the relative efficacy of these medications in GAD and panic disorder.

Justification for using antidepressants in GAD

Further justification for the use of antide-pressants in the treatment of DSM IV GAD comes from four sources. Wittchen et al found in the epidemiology catchment area (ECA) study that among patients presenting with GAD, 89.9% had at least one co-morbid axis I psychiatric disorder.[19] Of the co-morbid disorders, the most common was major depression in 62.4% of cases.[19] Strictly, the DSM IV criterion F states that GAD and major depression cannot coexist concurrently.[18] However, this is at variance with the observation that very often patients presenting with typical symptoms of GAD have major depression. Alcohol (37.6% of GAD patients) and drug abuse (27.6% of GAD patients) and other anxiety disorders are frequently co-morbid with GAD.[19] In such cases, antidepressants are preferable to benzodiazepines.

A study by Lecrubier and Hergueta (1998) found that patients identified by primary care physicians as having a mental health problem were much more likely to give an anxiety diagnosis than a depression diagnosis by an order of magnitude of three to one.[20] In contrast, an expert specialist using a struc-tured interview (the CIDI) with the same patients was more likely to give a depression than an anxiety disorder diagnosis.[20] The over-diagnosis of anxiety more or less offset the under-diagnosis of depression to give rates that match those by the expert specialist with a structured interview.[20] The implications of these findings is that if clinicians think they see an anxiety disorder, it is often likely to be depression and if they choose an anxiolytic to treat such a depressed patient the outcome will be disappointing.

A recent finding by Wittchen et al[21] showed the cumulative risk of later developing major depression was much higher for those diagnosed with GAD than for other anxiety disorders in aggregate. Therefore if we use an anxiolytic to treat today's GAD it will not adequately protect that patient from later developing depression. On the other hand, if we use an anxiolytic antidepressant to treat GAD today, it has a high likelihood of protecting that patient against subsequent major depressive episodes.

Data from the Collaborative Depression Study and the Harvard Anxiety Research Program datasets followed two cohorts of patients in the community longitudinally; one cohort with GAD and the other cohort with major depression.[22,23] Patients with major depression were more likely to have responded to treatment at 6 months (54% vs. 11%), 2 years (81% vs. 25 %) and 5 years (88% vs. 38%), than patients with GAD.[22,23] This is the opposite of what many clinicians expect. The reasons for this are not entirely clear. However, at the time of those analyses (1992), patients with major depression were treated mainly with antidepressants, while patients with GAD were mainly treated with anxiolytics like benzodiazepines or buspirone.[22,23] The relative lack of superior efficacy with benzodiazepines and buspirone compared to antidepressants in GAD may explain the relative failure of GAD patients to respond as well to treat-ment in the community as do patients with major depression.

Table 11.1 Studies of antidepressants in the treatment of generalized anxiety disorder

Author	Design	Test drug	N	Comparator	N	Wks	Result
Rickels et al [17]	DB, PC, FLD	Imipramine 143 mg Trazodone 255 mg	58 61	Diazepam 26 mg Placebo	56 55	8	Imipramine > Trazodone > Diazepam > Placebo
Hedges et al [35]	OL, FLD	Nefazodone 375 mg	21			8	Decrease in HAM-A
Rocca et al [31]	OL, FLD	Paroxetine 20 mg	30	Imipramine 75 mg Diazepam 4 mg	26 25	8	Paroxetine & Imipramine > Diazepam
Rickels et al [32]	DB, PC, FD	Paroxetine 20 mg 40 mg	189 197	Placebo	180	8	Both doses of Paroxetine > Placebo
Pollack et al [33]	DB, PC, FLD	Paroxetine 20–50 mg	162	Placebo	164	8	Paroxetine > Placebo mean dose 34.3 mg
Stocchi et al [34]	DB, PC, FLD	Paroxetine 20–50 mg	652 Single blind	Placebo	288	8 Single blind; 24 DB	Paroxetine > Placebo mean dose 28.4 mg
Davidson et al [26]	DB, PC, FD	Venlafaxine XR 75 mg 150 mg	87 87	Buspirone 30 mg Placebo	93 98	8	Venlafaxine > Buspirone > Placebo
Rickels et al [25]	DB, PC, FD	Venlafaxine XR 75 mg 150 mg 225 mg	86 81 86	Placebo	96	8	Venlafaxine > Placebo
Gelenberg et al [28]	DB, PC, FLD	Venlafaxine XR 75 to 225 mg	124	Placebo	127	24	Venlafaxine > Placebo
Allgulander et al [27]	DB, PC, FD	Venlafaxine XR 37.5 mg 75 mg 150 mg	138 130 131	Placebo	130	24	Venlafaxine 75 & 150 mg > Placebo. Venlafaxine 37.5 mg = placebo

Key: DB = Double blind; PC = placebo controlled; OL = open label; FLD = flexible dosing; fD = Fixed dose; Wks = weeks.

The investigation of SSRIs and SNRIs in the treatment of GAD

The newer antidepressants offer significant advantages over the tricyclics, monoamine oxidase inhibitors and other non-antidepressant medications. These advantages include the control of anxiety and co-morbid depression with the use of a single medicine, decreased risk of dependence or withdrawal symptoms, a more tolerable side effect profile, reduced interaction potential with alcohol and low lethality in overdose. All of these advantages suggest that one of the newer antidepressants be the first choice in treatment. Clinical experience suggests that all selective serotonin reuptake inhibitors (SSRIs) and the serotonin norepinephrine reuptake inhibitors (SNRIs) have efficacy in anxiety disorders though, as yet, only venlafaxine and paroxetine are licensed for GAD (see later). Paroxetine is licensed for the widest range of anxiety disorders (OCD, panic disorder, social anxiety disorder, GAD and PTSD) of all antidepressant therapies (see Table 11.2). However, there are differences in tolerability, safety and drug interactions. There are big differences in the scientific rigor and the extent to which each has been studied for regulatory approval across all the anxiety disorder indication (Table 11.1).

Although there are six SSRIs/SNRIs on the US market approved for at least one indication at the time of this writing (2002), only two of these have received FDA approval for both the short-term and longer term (6 months) treatment of GAD (venlafaxine XR and paroxetine). Double-blind placebo-controlled studies leading to FDA approval now appear highly unlikely either for fluoxetine, fluvoxamine or citalopram in their current formulations, since they are either off patent or about to go off patent before such studies can be done. A development program of GAD studies for an FDA indication is currently underway with sertraline and we await the results. In the

Table 11.2 Antidepressants approved by the FDA for the treatment of anxiety disorders

	PD	SAD	GAD	OCD	PTSD
Fluoxetine				X	
Sertraline	X			X	X
Paroxetine	X	X	X	X	X
Paroxetine CR	X				
Citalopram					
Fluvoxamine				X	
Venlafaxine			X		
Nefazadone					
Escitalopram					
Trazodone					
Mirtazapine					

PD = Panic disorder, SAD = social anxiety disorder, GAD = generalized anxiety disorder, OCD = obsessive compulsive disorder, PTSD = post traumatic stress disorder.

meantime, this does not preclude the use of other SSRIs such as sertraline, fluvoxamine, fluoxetine, or citalopram by clinicians when they feel it justified, but the FDA has not approved their use in GAD (Table 11.2). Currently, in the authors' opinion, paroxetine is the SSRI of choice in GAD based on the wealth of published data.

Venlafaxine XR

The first medication in the last decade to pursue a GAD indication was venlafaxine XR (sustained release formulation) in a dose range of 75–225 mg/d. Venlafaxine XR is a serotonin and norepinephrine reuptake inhibitor (SNRI). It also rapidly reduces ß-adrenergic receptor sensitivity in animal models, in comparison to other antidepressants.[24] Short[25,26] and long-term studies[27,28] of pure GAD, and of depression with comorbid anxiety[29] found venlafaxine XR was effective. Although equivalent mg for mg to venlafaxine IR, these doses are lower than the ceiling doses of 375 mg/d of venlafaxine IR (immediate release) studied in major depression. This does not mean that clinicians should never or will never need to use higher doses for patients with GAD. In our experience, this is sometimes necessary to provide a good treatment result. However, the scientific data supporting the use of such doses in GAD is not adequately studied nor FDA approved.

Four large multicenter, double-blind, placebo-controlled published studies investigated the effect of Venlafaxine XR in GAD. One was a flexible dose design, while three were fixed dose designs. All were for 8 weeks and used similar inclusion and exclusion criteria. In one study, buspirone (30 mg/d) was used as an active comparator. There were two 6-month studies (2-month acute phase followed by a 4-month continuation phase). One of these long-term studies was a fixed dose design while the other was a flexible dose design.

In an 8-week, double-blind, placebo-controlled study of DSM IV GAD without depression,[25] venlafaxine XR was significantly superior to placebo in lowering the HAM-A total score ($p<0.05$), including the HAM-A psychic anxiety factor ($p<0.01$) and on the Clinical Global Impression (CGI) global improvement and severity of illness scores ($p<0.05$).[25] It also showed superiority on the Hospital Anxiety and Depression scale (HAD) ($p<0.01$). The 225 mg dose was more effective than the 75 mg or 150 mg doses across the spectrum of all seven outcome measures used in the study and persisted through the end of the study.

In a study, comparing it to buspirone and placebo, venlafaxine XR (75 mg and 150 mg/day) was more effective than placebo in the HAM-A psychic factor ($p<0.05$) but in the HAM-A total only at a statistical trend level ($p<0.10$).[26] Patients on venlafaxine XR 75 mg showed a significantly superior response to buspirone and placebo on the CGI severity and CGI improvement ratings ($p<0.05$). Venlafaxine XR (75 mg and 150 mg/day) resulted in a significantly greater improvement than placebo or buspirone in the HAD anxiety sub-scale ($p<0.05$).[26]

A long-term study[27] over 24 weeks used doses of 37.5, 75 and 150 mg of venlafaxine XR or placebo.[27] Those on active drug at either 75 or 150 mg but not 37.5 mg showed response on the HAM-A, the HAD and the HAM-A psychic anxiety factor beyond that of placebo ($p<0.05$). Clinical improvement was better in the higher doses.

A second long-term double-blind flexible dose study compared venlafaxine XR (75–225 mg/day) to placebo over 28 weeks.[28] Dosage adjustments as clinically indicated were allowed.[28] The mean final dose of venlafaxine

XR was 176mg.[28] Patients on active drug showed significantly greater improvement (p<0.05) on the HAM-A, CGI, the HAD and Covi Anxiety Scale than those on placebo.[28] Venlafaxine XR separated statistically from placebo as early as week 1 of the study and remained superior to placebo through the end of the study.[28] However, the benefit was only clinically meaningful by the 4th week.[28]

Analysis of pooled data from the two long-term studies[30] showed that 66% of patients on venlafaxine XR met criteria for response (defined as ≥50% reduction from baseline in HAM-A total scores) and 43% for remission (defined as HAM-A≤7). For patients on placebo, the response rate was 38% (p<0.001) and the remission rate was 19% (p<0.001).[30] By week 8, more patients with moderate GAD severity (baseline HAM-A scores of 18–25) had achieved remission than those with severe GAD severity (baseline HAM-A >25).[30] However, by week 24 both the moderate and severe GAD groups had the same remission rates (43%).[30] This was not true for the patients on placebo where only 15–23% had achieved remission.[30] The clinical implication of this observation is that the more severely ill patients need more time to heal. However, given a long enough course of treatment the severe GAD patients have as good a chance of achieving remission as the moderately severe. This supports the recommendation that clinicians should be patient and not keep switching medications in the face of a partial response. Overall, in the venlafaxine XR group, 61% of those who had responded at week 8 went on to achieve remission, as compared to a 39% conversion rate in the placebo group.[30]

Paroxetine

Efficacy for paroxetine in GAD was first reported by Rocca et al.[31] They compared paroxetine to imipramine and chlordesmethy-diazepam using an open label, randomized design of 8 weeks' duration.[31] The daily dose of paroxetine was 20 mg, the mean daily dose of imipramine was 75 mg (range 50–100), and for the benzodiazepine was 4.2 mg (range 3–6 mg).[31] During the first 2 weeks of treatment, the maximum reduction in anxiety was observed in those patients treated with the benzodiazepine and from week 4 greater reductions were seen with those treated with antidepressants.[31] The benzodiazepine mainly influenced somatic anxiety symptoms while the antidepressants had a better impact on psychic anxiety symptoms.[31]

In the paroxetine drug development program for GAD, there were three large multi-centered 8-week double-blind placebo-controlled studies involving an aggregate of 1264 patients and one double-blind placebo-controlled relapse prevention study (8 weeks single blind paroxetine 20–50 mg/day treatment followed by double-blind randomization to paroxetine 20–50 mg/day or placebo for 24 weeks) in 652 patients. Of the short-term studies, one was a fixed dose design (20 and 40 mg/d; n = 566). The other two were flexible dose designs (dose range 20 to 50 mg/d; n = 326; n = 372).

• Paroxetine was studied in 566 patients with GAD over 8 weeks at fixed doses of 20 or 40 mg.[32] Both doses were superior to placebo in decreasing the HAM-A total score (p<0.001) and on the HAM-A anxiety and worry item (p<0.001). On Paroxetine 20 mg, the response rate (defined as patients achieving a CGI global impression score of 1 [very much improved] or 2 [much improved]) was 68% and on 40 mg it was 81%, the response for placebo was 52% these are OC data. LOCF data = 62% 20mg, 68% 40mg vs 46% placebo – statistically significantly different from placebo p<0.05 20mg vs placebo.[32] Remission rates (HAM-A ≤7) were 36% for Paroxetine 40 mg, 30% for the 20 mg dose and 20% for the placebo group[32]. Impairments in work, family, and social life (assessed using the Sheehan Disability Scale, SDS, items) improved significantly with paroxetine treatment (p<0.001) vs placebo.[32] These findings were replicated in the USA placebo controlled flexible dose study involving 326 patients treated over 8 weeks.[33] Paroxetine was significantly superior to placebo in decreasing the mean total HAM-A scores and the HAM-A items 1 and 2 (p<0.05 all endpoints). Statistically significant separation from placebo was observed as early as week 1 of the study on HAM-A item 1 [33]. The mean final effective dose of paroxetine was 34.3 mg/day.[33]

More recently, a 32-week relapse prevention study was undertaken to evaluate the long-term efficacy of paroxetine in 652 adult patients with GAD.[34] Statistically significant fewer paroxetine-treated patients relapsed compared with placebo (10.9% and 39.9%, respectively). Indeed, patients in the placebo group were approximately five times more likely to relapse than patients on continuous paroxetine treatment. There was also a significant difference in favour of paroxetine in time to relapse (p<0.001). Anxiety symptoms and functional disability continued to improve during long-term treatment with paroxetine.

Nefazodone

Nefazodone acts as an antagonist at 5-HT2A and 5-HT2c receptors and blocks 5-HT reuptake. It also blocks norepinephrine uptake, but this diminishes over time. M-chlorophenylpiperazine (mCPP) is a metabolite of nefazodone is also an agonist at the 5-HT2c receptor and may be anxiogenic. In an open label study,[35] nefazodone was used to treat 21 patients with GAD but no depression. Fifteen patients completed the study, 12 of them reported benefit in the reduction of anxiety symptoms on the HAM-A [35]. This finding has not yet been replicated in double blind placebo controlled studies.

Tolerability

In view of the need for long-term use of these medications, other considerations, in addition to efficacy, such as side effects, tolerability, and potential for drug interactions in the long term, are an important part of the risk benefit ratio. Nausea and headache with initial treatment is a common occurrence with all SSRIs. Activation and initial anxiety is more likely with fluoxetine, diarrhea with sertraline, nausea with fluvoxamine, sedation with nefazodone and paroxetine, sweating and small blood pressure elevations with venlafaxine XR. Very modest weight gain in some patients (1–4 kg over 1 year) is possible on all SSRIs long term, but whether there are weight gain differences among the SSRIs long term at doses that deliver remission is still a matter of vigorous debate and not supported by rigorous scientific evidence in spite of claims to the contrary. Sexual dysfunction, particularly delayed ejaculation or orgasm, occurs with all the SSRIs and SNRIs including citalopram, but is least problematic with nefazodone. Review of the aggregate evidence from several sources suggests that sexual side effects are equally likely with all the SSRIs, at adequate therapeutic doses, and that claims to the contrary are marketing hype not supported by compelling credible scientific data. These medications are inhibitors of hepatic

Table 11.3 Relative inhibition of CYP450 isoenzymes by serotonin re-uptake inhibitors				
	1A2	**2C19**	**2D6**	**3A4**
Fluoxetine	+	++	+++	++
Paroxetine	+		+++	+
Nefazodone	+		+	+++
Sertraline	+		+	+
Fluvoxamine	+++	+	+	+++
Citalopram			+	
Venlafaxine	+	+	+	+

Key: mild inhibition = +, moderate = ++, severe = +++.

cytochrome p450 isoenzymes. To this extent, many SSRIs drive up the blood levels of other medications metabolized by these isoenzymes. The 3A4 p450 isoenzyme system is the one involved in the metabolism of more medications than any other. The 2D6 system is of special interest to psychiatrists because it is involved in the metabolism of many tricyclics and neuroleptics. Clinicians need not over-react with alarm to this interaction potential but need to understand it, be properly informed and vigilant, and understand how to circumvent the associated problems. Table 11.3 shows the relative inhibition of these enzymes by the various SSRIs/SNRIs.

Antidepressants: where do they work best in GAD?

In a most revealing analysis of the effect of venlafaxine XR on each individual item on the Hamilton Anxiety Scale, Hackett and Meoni found a differential impact on the various symptom clusters in GAD.[36] They investigated the effect size over 6 months of treatment in a large sample on venlafaxine XR in a double-blind placebo-controlled study. Effect size reflects the power of the drug on each symptom cluster. The biggest impact of venlafaxine XR was in the area of worry, anxious mood, tension, and the clinician's observation that the patient was anxious. They noted the same effect on another little used scale – the BSA (the brief scale for anxiety) which has a specific worry item. The impact on these items was greater than the impact on a range of somatic anxiety symptom clusters. This finding is consistent with the earlier finding of Rickels et al that the biggest impact of antidepressants comes in the area of psychic anxiety (worry, anxious mood and tension), an area where the older anxiolytics have yielded relatively disappointing results. With the reformulation of GAD in DSM IV[18], it has become more a syndrome of worry and less somatically centered than in earlier diagnostic classifications.

With this in mind, we have found that the WAT scale (Figure 11.1) is a very sensitive outcome measure in GAD and a very sensitive discriminator between drug and placebo. Studies are underway to see if it outperforms the HAM-A in this regard. It is a simple, short, self-rated, and useful instrument in clinics to track response to treatment in GAD patients.

Remission is the goal of treatment

Measuring quality in service delivery and providing satisfaction to customers in service industries has always been a challenge. In the business world one agreed-on principle is that it is necessary to meet or exceed the customers' expectations of the service provided. Although other business sectors give much attention to this, it has received little attention in medical service delivery.

Please mark ONE circle for each scale.

WORRY

In the past week, how much have you suffered from worry?

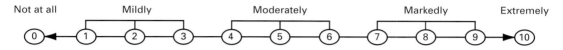

ANXIETY

In the past week, how much have you suffered from anxiety?

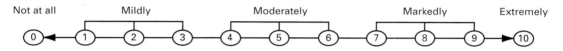

TENSION

In the past week, how much have you suffered from tension?

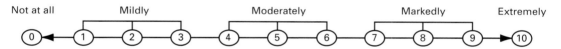

Figure 11.1 WAT (Worry–Anxiety–Tension): a brief, patient rated treatment outcome tracking scale for generalized anxiety dirsorder. ©2000 D. Sheehan. All rights reserved. Reproduced with permission.

With this in mind, we conducted a study to measure patients' expectations of an acceptable outcome, given that results might not be perfect.[37] The results revealed that the majority of anxious patients consistently reported that when they sought treatment they expected at least 70% or greater improvement.[37] Few settled for much less.[37] When outcomes fell short of 70% improvement patients said they were disappointed in both the clinician and the medication treatment. One of the authors (DS) has frequently polled psychiatrist audiences at lectures on their expectations of an acceptable (even if not perfect) outcome for their anxious or depressed patients. Consistently 70% is the level of improvement expert specialists expect from the treatments they use in their practices. There appears to be remarkable consistency in this 70% 'line in the sand' threshold that clinicians must deliver and patients expect from treatment, to meet or exceed expectations (see also Ballenger).[38,39]

With this in mind, it is surprising that results of treatment studies have until recently failed to report results of remission analysis publications on treatment studies – especially since this is what both patients and clinicians expect. The recent concept of remission embodies this 'need to improve 70% or more' outcome. Remission is defined in a variety of anxiety and mood disorders by anchoring it to a scale score on some symptom scale outcome measure, e.g. ≤ 7 on the HAM-A in GAD or ≤ 7 on the HAMD in depression. All these scores are anchored closely to this '70% rule of remission' across a range of disorders. Response, in contrast, is defined as a 50% improvement.

While the percentage of patients who meet this remission goal is much lower than that reported in responder analysis results, the data in remission analyses is much more consistent with clinicians' own clinical perceptions of results and treatment effects than information found in responder analysis. Indeed, researchers continue to be surprised at how revealing such remission analyses are. All pharmaceutical companies and researchers reporting results from treatment studies should now be encouraged to include such remission analyses in their reports (publications and slide sets). Regulatory agencies should pay more attention to this outcome threshold in evaluating treatment data. Clinicians setting goals for treatment outcomes should adopt this '$\geq 70\%$ rule' as a simple goal of treatment expectations across several domains of outcome and across all disorders. It would bring reports on studies in line with clinical expectations. Remission so defined, rather than response, is the goal of treatment.

We have found the 21 point Patient Global Improvement Scale to be a useful sensitive measure of improvement in our patients (see Figure 11.2). It also usefully anchors response, remission, and recovery. It may be more sensitive than the 50-year-old CGI that is used so frequently as an outcome measure in clinical trials.

The old CGI was not designed to discriminate sensitively between two active and effective medications in clinical trials. Results with the old CGI can give the impression that two effective medications are equally effective when they

How much has your condition improved or worsened since starting this study or treatment?

Please mark the circled number that rates your change copared to the start of the study or treatment.

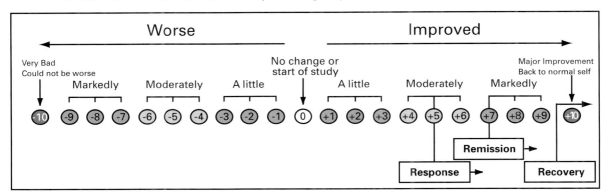

Figure 11.2 Patient Global Improvement Scale: a brief, patient-rated, treatment outcome tracking scale, with the aim of achieving at least 70% improvement.

are not. A more sensitive CGI should be better able to make such a distinction. This has implications for translating such research data into clinical practice recommendations.

Time to remission

What are the results of remission in GAD? A simple rule is that after 8 weeks of treatment between 40 and 50% of GAD patients in double-blind placebo-controlled studies with an ITT/LOCF analysis have met or exceeded remission threshold. The higher the dose within the usual therapeutic range, the greater the percentage of patients who achieve remission. Placebo achieves 15–25% remission rates under similar conditions.

In a recent study with paroxetine, Stocchi et al found that at week 1, 0.5% were in remission, at week 2, 3% and at week 3, 9.7%.[34] By week 8, 47.9% of patients were in remission and by week 32, 73% were in remission. Indeed, over the time frames in the longest studies ever carried out in GAD, the odds of converting into remission never stop increasing from each time point to the following visit. Patients are constantly moving from non-responsive to response and from response to remission over many months of treatment.

If patients are told that the medication/ treatment will 'help' them in '2 or 3 weeks' they hear 'I will be 70% or more improved in 2 to 3 weeks'. This only occurs in less than 10% of patients on SSRIs and SNRIs. The great majority falls short of this. It is therefore not surprising that many patients stop taking their medication before it delivers the benefits that are possible with time. We do our patients a favor if we inform them more accurately of the time to remission. This will set realistic expectations, enhance compliance, and lead to the patient respecting the clinician for their greater accuracy in predicting outcomes to match expectations.

Relapse and discontinuation

The relapse rate following discontinuation is considerable. In one recent GAD relapse prevention study, patients were treated for 2 months with 20–50 mg of single blind paroxetine to get the best therapeutic benefit for each patient.[34,40] After 2 months, those who responded entered into a double blind phase where they were randomized to either continue on the same dose of paroxetine or slowly tapered off onto placebo.[34,40] The risk of full relapse was assessed over the next 6 months;[34] 10.9% had a full relapse during this time on paroxetine while 39.9% relapsed fully on placebo.[34,40] These differences were statistically significant (p<0.001).[34,40] Clinical experience suggests that when effective antidepressant treatments for GAD are stopped a proportion of patients have partial relapses and want to restart their medication to prevent further deterioration.

Many of the anxiolytics, including several of the best-studied antidepressant anxiolytics (e.g. venlafaxine XR and paroxetine), have short half-lives. Withdrawal reactions have been described for all SSRIs and SNRIs even those with longer half-lives. With a longer half-life medication, the time until emergence of withdrawal symptoms is much longer, at which point many do not make a connection between the discontinuation of the medication and the emergent withdrawal symptoms. They may even blame the new medication they have started for these symptoms. Because abrupt discontinuation can result in more disruptive withdrawal symptoms, especially if the patient has been on the medication for a long time, they should always be withdrawn very, very slowly i.e. over weeks rather than days. For example, we taper paroxetine and citalopram at a rate of no faster than 10 mg every 4 to 7 days (or 25 mg of sertraline or 75 mg of venlafaxine). At such rates taper takes at least 2 weeks or longer to complete. Withdrawal reactions observed following discontinuation of SSRIs and SNRIs are not medically dangerous, but are subjectively unpleasant. A slow taper schedule can minimize this problem.

Dosing strategies

In practice, physicians use different dosing strategies when using antidepressants. Some dose to a specific number of milligrams. They learn a dose for each antidepressant they use and start the patient off on a standard size tablet or capsule. They wait and hope this will provide the desired benefit within a few weeks. If not, they try a second antidepressant using a similar strategy. If two such trials fail they may send the patient to a specialist.

Many specialists prefer a different strategy – to titrate the dose until they get a therapeutic effect. Depending on their expectations of outcome, their comfort with the medication and their concern about side effects, this strategy may be effective or may deliver less than ideal results. Some specialists use rating scales to guide them in anchoring outcome to a scale score, much as physicians use lab test results to track outcome in medical illnesses. However, this strategy, although both desirable and commendable, can prolong time to achieve a good result.

Many experienced psychopharmacologists titrate to side effects rather than to an a priori mg dose. If there are no side effects, they consider this dose will not provide the optimal benefit. This strategy is often the most reliable, efficient, rapid and effective way to provide the best therapeutic results especially in difficult cases. To implement this strategy correctly,

start at the lowest possible dose and increase the dose up in very small increments very, very slowly. For example, if the tablet size of an antidepressant is 20 mg (e.g., paroxetine, fluoxetine or citalopram), start with half a tablet (10 mg) after the evening meal. For sertraline, we start with half a 50 mg tablet and with venlafaxine start with 37.5 mg. We keep the patient on this dose for a full week. If patients are instructed to take the dose first thing in the morning, they are likely to skip breakfast and to take the dose on an empty stomach and then to wash the tablet down with a few cups of coffee. This is often disruptive. It is usually preferable to take the medication either after the evening meal or at bedtime. Other clinicians are slightly more aggressive in the dosing of their anxious patients.

With SSRIs, the side effects that are in our opinion the best guide to the optimal therapeutic dose are the presence of mild nausea and mild headaches (not vomiting or crushing migraine). If there are no side effects at the end of each week, increase the dose by a half tablet (another 10 mg) after the evening meal. We repeat this weekly until the onset of mild nausea/queasiness and/or mild frontal headaches. We hold the dose at this level and do not lower it unless these side effects are too disruptive to the patient. The patient is encouraged to hold the dose at this level over the following week. Typically, the nausea and headaches subside within 4 to 7 days of their onset. Usually, this dose will provide the optimal therapeutic effect 4 to 6 weeks later and is the dose that is more likely to protect the patient in the long run against future recurrences. This strategy calls for a slow, gentle, but relentless dose increase in pursuit of the dose that provides the best chance of remission.

When the patient has achieved remission, we do not lower the dose down to a 'maintenance level' of half that amount. To lower the dose below that required to achieve remission is to invite a risk of recurrence. There is no such thing as a 'maintenance dose' of an antidepressant. The maintenance dose is in the full effective therapeutic dose that provided remission in the first place.

Medication strategy

Figure 11.3 captures the medication strategy that is now most widely used in the treatment of GAD. We first start patients presenting with GAD on either an SNRI or an SSRI. We increase the dose as outlined above over several weeks. We keep them on the optimal therapeutic dose for at least 8 to 10 weeks. If they reach remission on this dose, we keep them on this medication for at least one year. Studies have shown that some patients, particularly those with high anxiety levels, may take as long as 6 months to achieve remission. If there is only a partial response after 4 to 6 weeks of treatment, the clinician should be patient and not switch to another antidepressant too soon. Some very anxious patients may require the addition of an anxiolytic in the early weeks of treatment while waiting for a good response to the antidepressant. Once the patient achieves remission, treatment should continue for at least 1 year. After a year, we review the wisdom of tapering. In some patients, it may be prudent to treat for even longer periods. If a patient had three or more episodes of GAD in their lifetime, it may be wiser to stay on the medication long term to protect them against future recurrences (see Ballenger et al).[41]

If the patient does not reach remission or at least a significant improvement within a reasonable time (e.g. 8–10 weeks), this is an unsatisfactory response. Consider switching the patient over to another SSRI or to an SNRI or a serotonin antagonist reuptake inhibitor or an MAO inhibitor or an anticonvulsant like sodium valproate (Figure 11.3). Other options include a benzodiazepine, buspirone, hydroxyzine, cognitive behaviour therapy or psychotherapy. Use each of these for trials of 8 to 10 weeks squeezing the dose up to the maximum level the patient can tolerate and always coming back to the central question, 'how well has the patient recovered?' If they have reached remission, keep them on the medication at that dose for at least a year. At that point, review the wisdom of tapering. Many more patients are going to require long-term medication management than we were willing to admit in the past if we are to protect the patient from relapse and further disability. If they have not recovered well enough after 8 to 10 weeks they should then be moved on to the next medication in the series (Figure 11.3). Repeat this until you find the medication and appropriate dose that delivers the most satisfactory outcome. These treatment alternatives may include tricyclic antidepressants, buspirone, the benzodiazepines or augmentation strategies with either a second anxiolytic/antidepressant or some type of psychotherapy.

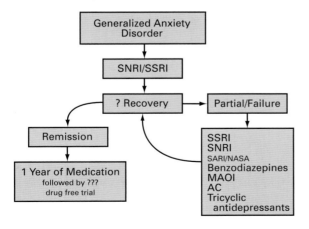

Figure 11.3 Medication strategy. ©1995 D. Sheehan. All rights reserved. Reproduced with permission.

Summary and take home message

An accumulation of data suggests that SSRIs and the SNRIs (especially paroxetine and venlafaxine) are very effective in GAD, not only in the acute treatment but also in the long-term treatment and in relapse prevention (though currently only paroxetine has demonstrated effectiveness in relapse prevention). They are particularly effective in targeting the core GAD symptoms of worry, anxious mood, and tension. In addition, they improve the work disability, social life disability and family life disability associated with GAD. Rate of remission increases with length of therapy.

The take home message is that the best treatment for GAD is no longer an anxiolytic, but rather one of the newer SSRI/SNRI antidepressants.

References

1. The American Psychiatric Association, Diagnostic and Statistical Manual of Mental Disorders (3rd edition, DSM-III) (1980) Washington, DC.

2. Fontaine R, Mercier P, Beaudry P et al, Bromazepam and lorazepam in generalized anxiety: a placebo-controlled study with measurement of drug plasma concentrations, *Acta Psychiatr Scand* (1986) 75: 451–8.

3. Fontaine R, Annable L, Chouinard G, Ogilvie R, Bromazepam and diazepam in generalized anxiety: a placebo controlled study with measurement of drug plasma concentrations, *J Clin Psychopharmacol* (1983) 3: 80–87.

4. Rickels K, Csanalosi I, Greisman P et al, A controlled clinical trial of alprazolam for the treatment of anxiety, *Am J Psychiatry* (1983) 140: 82–5.

5. Bertin I, Colombo G, Furlanut M, Benetello, Double blind placebo cross over study of long acting (chlordesmethyldiazepam) versus short acting (lorazepam) benzodiazepines in generalized anxiety disorders, *Int J Clin Pharmacol Res* (1989) 9: 203–8.

6. Cutler NR, Sramek JJ, Hesselink JMK et al, A double blind, placebo controlled study comparing the efficacy and safety of ipsapirone versus lorazepam in patients with generalized anxiety disorder: A prospective multicenter trial, *J Clin Psychopharmacol* (1993) 13: 429–37.

7. Klein DF, Importance of psychiatric diagnosis and prediction of clinical drug effects, *Arch Gen Psychiatry* (1967) 16: 118–26.

8. Sheehan DV, Overcoming anxiety attacks and phobias: a patient's guide, *Drug Therapy* (1982) 12: 67–72.

9. Sheehan DV, Coleman JH, Greenblatt DJ et al, Some biochemical correlates of panic attacks with agoraphobia and their response to a new treatment, *J Clin Psychopharmacol* (1984) 4: 66–75.

10. Sheehan DV, Claycomb, JB, Surman OS, The relative efficacy of alprazolam, phenelzine and imipramine in treating panic attacks and phobias, *Abstracts of 137th Annual meeting of the American Psychiatric Association* (1984) 83.

11. Chouinard G, Annable L, Fontaine R et al, Alprazolam in the treatment of generalized anxiety and panic disorders: a double blind placebo controlled study, *Psychopharmacology* (1982) 77: 229–33.

12. Ballenger JC, Burrows, GD, Dupont RL, Alprazolam in panic disorder and agoraphobia: results from a multicenter trial: efficacy in short-term treatment, *Arch Gen Psychiatry* (1988) 45: 413–22.

13. Katschnig H, Amering M, Stolk JM et al, Long-term follow-up after a drug trial for panic disorder, *Br J Psychiatry* (1995) 167: 487–94.

14. Rickels K, Csanalosi I, Greisman et al, A controlled clinical trial of alprazolam for the treatment of anxiety, *Am J Psychiatry* (1983) 140: 82–5.

15. Sheehan DV, Raj BA, Harnett-Sheehan K, et al, Adinazolam sustained release formulation in the treatment of generalized anxiety disorder. *J Anxiety Disord* (1990) 4: 239–46.

16. Sheehan DV, Raj BA, Harnett-Sheehan K et al, Adinazolam sustained release formulation in the treatment of panic disorder. *Irish J Psychol Med* (1990) 7: 124–8.

17. Rickels K, Downing R, Schweizer E, Hassman H, Antidepressants for the treatment of generalized anxiety disorder. A placebo-controlled comparison of imipramine, trazodone and diazepam, *Arch Gen Psychiatry* (1993) 50: 884–95.

18. American Psychiatric Association, Diagnostic and Statistical Manual of Mental Disorders (4th ed., DSM-IV) (1994) Washington, DC.

19. Wittchen H-U, Zhao S, Kessler RC, Eaton WW, DSM-111-R Generalized Anxiety Disorder in the National Comorbidity Survey, *Arch Gen Psychiatry* (1994) **51**: 355–64.

20. Lecrubier Y, Hergueta T, Differences between prescription and consumption of antidepressants and anxiolytics, *Int Clin Psychopharmacol* (1998) **13**(Suppl 2): S7–11.

21. Wittchen H-U, Presentation on 'Epidemology and Clinical Features of Generalized Anxiety Disorder' at workshop on 'Controversies, Challenges and Consensus in Generalized Anxiety Disorder, 15th Collegium Internationale of Neuropsychopharmacologium Congress (CINP) Brussels, Belgium, July 11, 2000

22. Coryell W, Endicott J, Keller M, Outcome of patients with chronic affective disorder: a five year follow up, *Am J Psychiatry* (1990) **147**: 1627–33.

23. Keller, M Presentation on 'Longitudinal Course of Generalized Anxiety Disorder' at workshop on 'Controversies, Challenges and Consensus in Generalized Anxiety Disorder', 15th Collegium Internationale of Neuropsychopharmacologium Congress (CINP) Brussels, Belgium July 11, 2000

24. Mendlewicz J, Pharmacologic profile and efficacy of venlafaxine, *Int Clin Psychopharmacol* (1995) **10**(Suppl 2): 5–13.

25. Rickels K, Pollack MH, Sheehan DV, Haskins JT, Efficacy of venlafaxine extended release in nondepressed outpatients with generalized anxiety disorder, *Am J Psychiatry* (2000) **157**: 968–74.

26. Davidson JRT, Dupont RL, Hedges D, Haskins JT, Efficacy, safety and tolerability of venlafaxine extended release and buspirone in outpatients with generalized anxiety disorder, *J Clin Psychiatry* (1999) **60**: 528–35.

27. Allgulander C, Hackett D, Salinas E, Venlafaxine extended release (ER) in the treatment of Generalized Anxiety Disorder: twenty-four-week placebo-controlled dose-ranging study. *Br J Psychiatry* (2001) **179**: 15–22.

28. Gelenberg AJ, Lydiard RB, Rudolph RL et al, Efficacy of venlafaxine extended release capsules in nondepressed outpatients with generalized anxiety disorder, *JAMA* (2000) **283**: 3082–8.

29. Gorman JM, Papp LA, Efficacy of venlafaxine in mixed depression-anxiety states, *Depress Anxiety* (2000) **12**(Suppl 1): 77–80.

30. Montgomery SA, Sheehan DV, Meoni P, Haudiquet V, Hackett D, A 6-month trial: characterization of the longitudinal course of improvement in generalized anxiety disorder during long term treatment with Effexor XR (Venlafaxine HCL). Poster presentation, US Psychiatric Congress, 11/17/01, Boston, USA.

31. Rocca P, Fonzo V, Scotta M, Zanalda E, Ravizza L, Paroxetine efficacy in the treatment of generalized anxiety disorder, *Acta Psychiatr Scand* (1997) **95**: 444–50.

32. Rickels K, Zaninelli R, McCafferty J et al, Paroxetine treatment of generalized anxiety disorder: a double blind, placebo controlled trial. *Am J Psychiatry* in press

33. Pollack M, Zaninelli R, Goddard A et al, Paroxetine in the treatment of generalized anxiety disorder: results of a placebo controlled, flexible dosage trial. *J Clin Psychiatry* (2001) **62**: 350–57.

34. Stocchi F, Nordera G, Jokinen R, Lepola U, Efficacy and tolerability of paroxetine for long-term treatment of GAD, Poster presented at American Psychiatric Association (APA) 2001 Annual Meeting, New Orleans, LA, (2000). May 5–10, [abstract] NR635:171.

35. Hedges DW, Reimherr FW, Strong RE, Halls CH, Rust C, An open trial of nefazodone in adult patients with generalized anxiety disorder. *Psychopharmacol Bull* (1996) **32**: 671–6.

36. Hackett D, Meoni P Poster at American Psychiatric Association Meeting, New Orleans, LA 2001.

37. Sheehan DV. Why sustained-release medications? Practical considerations in the management of patients with anxiety. *Psychiatr Ann* (1993) (Suppl): 3–7.

38. Ballenger JC, Clinical guidelines for establishing remission in patients with depression and anxiety. *J Clin Psychiatry* (1999) **60** (Suppl 22): 29–34.

39. Ballenger JC, Treatment of anxiety disorders to remission. *J Clin Psychiatry* (2001) **62** (Suppl 12): 5–9.

40. Sheehan DV Presentation on 'Current Concepts in the diagnosis and treatment of Generalized Anxiety Disorder' at American Psychiatric Association Annual Meeting New Orleans, LA (2000).

41. Ballenger JC, Davidson JR, Lecrubier Y et al, Consensus statement on generalized anxiety disorder from the International Consensus Group on Depression and Anxiety. *J Clin Psychiatry* (2001) **62** (Suppl 11): 53–8.

IV   Special situations

12

Generalized Anxiety Disorder in Children and Adolescents

Moira A Rynn and Martin Franklin

Introduction

Generalized anxiety disorder (GAD) not only occurs across all ages but also is underdiagnosed at all developmental stages. Children with this diagnosis are often described as "little adults", often worrying about issues like finances, schedules, health of parents, future success, natural disasters, and safety. These children may not be disruptive in class or at home. Often, their internal distress is not noticed by adults who care for them. Alternatively, this distress may be expressed through physical symptoms such as headaches, stomachaches, insomnia, temper tantrums, heart palpitations, and dry mouth.

This disorder is highly comorbid with other childhood anxiety disorders such as separation anxiety disorder and social phobia. The studies described in this chapter treated children who had at least the diagnosis of GAD. In addition, symptomatology may change over time; a child may start with one anxiety disorder which later evolves into another primary anxiety disorder. Separation anxiety disorder is characterized by the child focusing on concerns about the safety of his or her parents or other family members, along with physical symptoms; for a diagnosis, cognitive and physical symptoms need to be present for at least four weeks. Socially phobic children report that their primary worry is embarrassing themselves in front of their peers or adults and experiencing this in social situations. The child with GAD may have these specific concerns, but they tend to possess worries in multiple domains of function.

Epidemiology

Defining the diagnosis

In the DSM-IIIR, there were three anxiety disorders that could be diagnosed in children and adolescents: overanxious disorder, separation anxiety disorder, and avoidant disorder. Overanxious disorder (OAD) has been removed from the DSM-IV, and children are now being diagnosed with generalized anxiety disorder (GAD). Overanxious and generalized anxiety disorder share most features.[1] Avoidant disorder has been removed, most likely due to its low prevalence and overlap with social phobia. Separation anxiety disorder is still listed in the section entitled 'Disorders Usually First Diagnosed in Infancy, Childhood and Adolescence'. Excessive anxiety and worry in a variety of areas that the child finds difficult to control characterize GAD.

Prevalence

Anxiety disorders, especially overanxious disorder and social phobia, are among the most common diagnoses reported in childhood and adolescent epidemiological studies.[2,3,4] Prevalence rates reported below for the childhood disorders are based on the diagnosis of overanxious disorder given the change to GAD with the DSM-IV. In community epidemiological studies, the prevalence rates for overanxious disorder have ranged from 2.9 to 4.6% and rates for separation anxiety disorder have ranged from 2.4 to 4.1%,[5-7] with 8.9% of a pediatric sample meeting criteria for any anxiety disorder.[7] Kashani and Orvaschel[8] in an adolescent sample reported prevalence rates of 17.3% for any anxiety disorder, 7.3% for overanxious disorder, and 7.0% for separation anxiety disorder. However, social withdrawal that interferes with functioning as evidenced by anxiety, isolation, hypersensitivity, depression, and self-consciousness has been reported in 10 to 20% of school-aged children[9,10]. Prevalence rates for internalizing disorders are higher in clinical samples, with 14% of patients being diagnosed with an anxiety disorder[11].

Impact

Because fears and anxieties are a normal part of development, they warrant attention and treatment only when they significantly inter-fere with academic, social, or interpersonal functioning or the mastery of developmental milestones. Children with anxiety disorders struggle with low self-esteem, social isolation, and inadequate social skills.[12] Anxiety's negative impact on social adjustment[13] and academic work[14] has been documented. In addition to impairment in functioning, children with anxiety disorders also frequently suffer from physical problems such as headaches, stomachaches, and irritable bowel syndrome,[15] leading to increased pediatrician visits and medical costs.

Although specific rates for GAD leading to school refusal are not known, worries and fears are estimated to contribute to 1.7% to 5.4% of school refusal cases.[16] The long-term consequences for school-refusing children include reduced opportunity for higher education, limited employment options, marital problems, social isolation, delinquency, and elevated risk for the development of psychiatric disorders.[16-20]

Phenomenology

There is growing evidence that childhood anxiety disorders and symptoms are not transitory but persist over time.[11,21,22] A recent school-based prevention trial by Dadds et al.[23] found that 54% of untreated children identified by self report and/or teachers' ratings with features of, but not the full diagnosis of an anxiety disorder developed an anxiety disorder over the 6 months of the study's monitoring period. In addition, older anxiety disordered children report significantly higher levels of anxiety (and depression) than younger children with the same diagnosis, suggesting that symptoms may worsen over time.[12] Children with overanxious disorder are likely to have other anxiety disorders at the same time.[24] However, a recent prospective study by Last et al.[25] suggests a more complex picture. Children with anxiety disorders were more likely than controls to develop new psychiatric disorders, primarily new anxiety disorders which was found over the 3 to 4-year follow-up phase of the study.

There also seems to be a link between childhood and adult manifestations of anxiety disorders. Many adults with anxiety disorders report suffering from separation anxiety or overanxious disorders as children.[26–28] One of the few prospective studies to have assessed anxious children's adjustment to early adulthood suggests that anxious children, especially those with comorbid depression, were less likely than controls (no history of psychiatric illness) to be living independently, to be working, or to be in higher education as adults.[29] Anxious children were also more likely to report psychological problems and to seek out mental health services in adulthood. Therefore, early intervention for these disorders may have profound implications both for altering the course of the disorder and for later adult development.

Inheritance

A number of studies have looked at the rates of anxiety and other psychiatric disorders in children of parents with anxiety disorders. Although less research has been conducted on the anxiety disorders compared to the depressive disorders, a limited number of twin and family studies has suggested that certain types of anxiety disorders may run in families.[30–33] Concordance for monozygotic twins was higher than for dizygotic twins for all anxiety disorders except generalized anxiety disorder,[30–33] which suggests that a predisposition for anxiety disorders may be transmitted genetically.

Family history studies have included direct clinical interviews of the children of parents with diagnosed disorders and have often compared parents who have anxiety and depressive disorders with a control group.[34–37] Children of parents with an anxiety disorder were found to be seven times more likely to receive an anxiety diagnosis than were children of controls, and twice as likely to receive an anxiety diagnosis than offspring of parents with dysthymic disorder.[35]

Examining specific anxiety disorders, Silverman et al.[38] had children of parents diagnosed with agoraphobia with panic, generalized anxiety disorder, panic disorder, and mixed phobias complete a structured interview and self-report measures. The parent was interviewed about the child and completed the Child Behavior Checklist (CBCL). Fifty percent of boys and 72% of girls of anxiety-disordered parents were found to have behavioral problems based on parental rating or interview. All clinical diagnoses were anxiety disorders. Analysing by parent diagnosis, 81% of children of agoraphobics, 75% of children of parents with mixed phobias, 29% of children of generalized anxiety disordered patients, but none of the children of panic disordered parents, received a clinical diagnosis and/or CBCL score in clinical range.

This evidence does suggest familial transmission, which may have implications for treatment.

Comorbidity

The high comorbidity rate of 30% for a co-occurrence of a depressive disorder for children in outpatient settings who have a diagnosis of an anxiety disorder points to the need to develop treatments for these disorders.[39] In addition, there is some evidence that as many as 41% of children or adolescents who suffer from major depression had or have an anxiety disorder that preceded the depression.[39,40] The presence of an anxiety disorder was found to lead to a worse prognosis for the depression, and at times had an effect on the length or recovery from the depressive episode. The anxiety disorder usually remained after treatment of and recovery from the depression.[40] Therefore treatment of the anxiety disorders may help in prevention of, or influence the course of, depressive disorders.

With different age groups, low to moderate comorbidity rates also exist for GAD and non-anxiety-related diagnoses. Younger children more often received a concurrent separation anxiety disorder (SAD) or attention deficit hyperactivity disorder (ADHD) diagnosis, whereas older children more often had concurrent simple phobia or major depression.[24,39] Several studies examined the comorbidity rates of depression and OAD, with rates ranging from 9 to 33%.[6,27,39] Kendall and colleagues[41] reported a comorbidity rate of 6% for anxiety disorders and depression in a randomized child clinical trial. Also commonly comorbid with primary OAD/GAD diagnoses are oppositional disorders.[27] It is clear that comorbidity dominates the clinical picture. It is more common for a child identified as having GAD to be comorbid with other diagnoses than it is for them to receive the single diagnosis.

Assessment

When assessing a child for anxiety disorders the clinician should be aware of several issues. First, the clinician should be aware of normal developmental childhood fears: some fear and anxiety is normal, and normal fear and anxiety in children has been well documented.[42] Second, there must be sensitivity to cultural and gender issues in assessment.[43–45] In addition, children differ from adults cognitively, and may have difficulty answering complex emotion-related questions.[46] Development of specific cognitive and language skills, as well as an understanding of self, emotions, and the perception of others will determine the adequacy of the interview.[46]

A detailed medical and family history should be obtained, as well as laboratory measures as indicated. For example, if the child complains of heat intolerance with warm, moist skin, weight loss, and rapid heart rate, it would be reasonable to do baseline thyroid studies. The treating clinician, with the consent of parent and child, should consult with the child's primary care physician to find out about any additional medical issues, and to check that the child has had a recent physical exam. This will also build collaboration with the primary care physician, who will support the treatment being recommended to the family.

Outlined below are several assessment instruments that will assist in establishing the type of anxiety the child is experiencing and how impairing it is for the child. Some of these instruments also take into account parental report. There are additional scales that are useful, and for a full description please refer to the review article by March & Albano.[47]

Assessment instruments

Clinician structured exam (Table 12.1)
Anxiety Disorders Interview Schedule for Children – Revised (ADIS-R)[48]
This is a clinical structured interview used to identify the principal diagnosis. This is operationally defined as the disorder associated with the most severe current and/or distress impairment, with the 0–8 distress/impairment sever-

ity scale. It is a revision of the original ADIS for DSM-IIIR.[38] This structured interview (which is based on Diagnostic and Statistical Manual of Mental Disorders, 4th edition) contains an expanded anxiety section not found in other available instruments, and also allows the assessor to screen for other disorders. The instrument requires screening for and the ability to diagnose all anxiety disorders (adult and child), affective disorders, as well as attention deficit disorder, oppositional disorder, conduct disorders and psychosis. The ADIS has satisfactory test-retest reliability[49,50] and moderate to high inter-rater reliability.[38,51] An illustration of its reliability and validity with a clinical sample can be found in Kendall[52] and Kendall et al.[41] The child and parent are interviewed separately and each provide a severity rating for each anxiety symptom on a scale of 0–8. This instrument is clearly written, directs the clinician on how to ask the questions, and assists with determining the diagnosis. This scale can be used throughout treatment to measure improvement.

Child self reports
The Multidimensional Anxiety Scale for Children (MASC)
This is a relatively new 39-item self report measure of anxiety in children (ages 8–18) that has four factors: physical symptoms, social anxiety, harm avoidance, and separation anxiety. March et al.[53] have provided internal consistency and test-retest reliability data. In addition, the scale has shown some promise to differentiate depression from anxiety in that it is not as highly correlated with the CDI as other anxiety measures. The factors mirror the DSM-IV diagnostic categories, and potentially the MASC could differentiate the symptoms of avoidance and physical complaints in anxiety. This scale can be given throughout treatment as another measure of clinical improvement.

The Revised Children's Manifest Anxiety Scale (RCMAS)[54]
This consists of 37 true/false items (28 anxiety and 9 Lie scale items) that assess a variety of anxiety symptoms.

Parent and teacher scale
Child Behavior Checklist (CBCL)[55,56]
The CBCL-P and T assess an array of behavioral problems and social competencies on a 0 to 2 point scale. The checklist provides scores on several specific behavioral problems as well as an overall internalizing and externalizing score. The specific factors vary with child's age and gender and are therefore reported as T scores to allow comparison of scores. Another section includes information on the child's functioning in a number of important domains (e.g. school, participation in social activities). The CBCL is widely used because of its reliability, validity, and established norms for both normal and clinical populations.[55,56] In addition, the CBCL includes items that can form a separate anxiety score (CBCL-Anxiety Scale[41]). This is completed by the parent and teacher at the initial evaluation, which provides information about the child's social function and behavior (age range 4–16 years).

Treatment

As mentioned earlier, many of the studies examining treatments include children and adolescents diagnosed with GAD, SAD, and SP, since these three anxiety diagnoses are frequently comorbid and overlapping in children. These anxiety disorders share an underlying construct of anxiety, exhibit strong association with each other, and frequently occur in comorbid state.

Table 12.1 Assessments

Assessment Scales	Descriptions
Anxiety Disorders Interview Schedule for Children – Revised (ADIS-R)	a. Clinician administered b. Semi-structured c. Takes about an hour and a half to complete d. All childhood disorders are covered and the clinician can choose to do only the sections that apply e. Severity/impairment scale is used to rate symptoms from 0 to 8
The Multidimensional Anxiety Scale for Children (MASC)	a. Child self report b. Takes the child about 20 mins to complete c. 39-item self report measure of anxiety in children (ages 8–18) that taps four factors: physical symptoms, social anxiety, harm avoidance, and separation anxiety d. Can be used to assess change of symptoms over time
The Revised Children's Manifest Anxiety Scale (RCMAS)	a. Child self report b. Takes the child about 15 mins to complete c. Consists of 37 true/false items (28 anxiety and 9 Lie scale items)
Child Behavior Checklist (CBCL)	a. Parent and teacher report b. The checklist provides scores on several specific behavioral problems as well as an overall internalizing and externalizing score c. The CBCL includes items that can form a separate anxiety score

The main treatments examined for these disorders are cognitive behavioral therapy and medications (primarily selective serotonin re-uptake inhibitors – SSRIs). Both treatments have demonstrated equal efficacy in adults and in children.[57,58] Both the parent and child need to be informed about the risks and benefits of treatment, and informed consent must be obtained prior to initiating treatment. It is important to be clear with the child and parent about what target symptoms will be monitored to determine treatment effectiveness.

Pharmacological treatment

Medication options for the treatment of GAD in children and adolescents include the benzodiazepines, the non-benzodiazepine anxiolytic buspirone, and the SSRI and tricyclic antidepressants.

Benzodiazepines
The benzodiazepines bind to the γ-aminobutyric acid (GABA) receptor membrane chloride channel complexes, which leads to enchanced central nervous system inhibition through the neurotransmitter GABA. Besides

their anxiolytic affect, benzodiazepines are also used for their anticonvulsant, hypnotic, and muscle relaxant properties.[59] Although there exists an extensive literature on the effectiveness of benzodiazepines in adult anxiety disorders,[60–62] there have been only a few studies, with small sample sizes, to examine the use of benzodiazepines in childhood anxiety disorders.[63,64] The majority of the studies involve children and adolescents with additional comorbidities such as major depression, panic disorder, and school refusal.[65,66] Biederman and colleagues[67] treated three prepubertal children who presented with panic symptoms, plus each had one additional anxiety disorder (separation anxiety disorder, avoidant disorder, or overanxious disorder). The children were treated with clonazepam, two with 0.5 mg/day and one with 3 mg/day, with positive results and no side effects. Simeon et al.[64] enrolled 30 patients, 8 to 16 years of age, with a primary diagnosis of overanxious disorder or avoidant disorder in a double-blind placebo-controlled study for four weeks treated with alprazolam. There was improvement in the patients on alprazolam (88%) as compared to placebo (62%); however, this difference was not statistically significant.

The most common side effects from benzodiazepines are drowsiness, headache, nausea, and fatigue. The side effects are dose-related and can lead to tremor, slurred speech, and ataxia.[62,68] There have been reports of "paradoxical reactions" in which the child experiences overexcitement, irritability, and perceptual disorganization. Another concern is the potential risk of dependence and withdrawal associated with the benzodiazepines, which rules them out as a front-line treatment. It is reasonable to assume that children could develop symptoms of dependence similar to those experienced by adults in terms of duration and type of withdrawal

symptoms. In our clinical experience benzodiazepines are useful as adjunct treatment with moderate to severe physical symptoms of anxiety, particularly when these interfere with the child attending school. It is recommended that if children and adolescents are treated with benzodiazepines that it is for a limited amount of time and at the lowest possible dose and, as clinically indicated. Once treatment is completed, the benzodiazepine should be gradually tapered to avoid the risk of withdrawal symptoms, such as insomnia, gastrointestinal complaints, rebound anxiety, and concentration difficulties.[69–71]

Although not recommended as a first choice of treatment, benzodiazepines may be effective for the child experiencing severe physical symptoms that may be contributing to his/her functional impairment, and they can serve as a useful adjunct for the first two weeks of antidepressant or psychosocial treatment.

Buspirone

Buspirone, a partial agonist at the serotonin 5-HT1A receptor, is a nonbenzodiazepine anxiolytic. Although it has been shown to have both anxiolytic and antidepressant effects in adults,[62,68] buspirone does not appear to be a highly effective or broad-spectrum anxiolytic in adults;[72,73] it does not appear to be a first choice for treatment with children. There is some evidence of improvement in open label trials.[70,74] Common side effects are headache, nausea, and dizziness.[75] The recommended dosage for children is 0.2 to 0.6 mg three times a day and for adolescents 5 to 10 mg three times a day with 5 to 10 mg increases every four days to the maximum dose of 60 mg per day.[76] There is no evidence of withdrawal with this medication, and its effects should be seen within six weeks.

Tricyclic antidepressants

The development of GAD may be due to the dysregulation of both the noradrenergic and serotonin system of the central nervous system. In general, the tricyclic antidepressants' (TCAs') therapeutic effectiveness in GAD is through the metabolism and/or the reuptake of the monoamine neurotransmitters.[59] The significant and often hard to tolerate side effects are due to the TCAs' blockade at the muscarinic/cholinergic, histamine (H1), and α-adrenergic receptors. The most common side effects are constipation, nausea, orthostatic hypotension, sedation, and weight gain.[77] The majority of clinical trials performed using TCAs did not feature children and adolescents with GAD only, but rather the more complicated comorbid group of school-refusing children. The several placebo-controlled studies of TCAs for school refusal have provided conflicting results.[65,78,79] Klein and colleagues[80] studied 20 children diagnosed with separation anxiety disorder who received either placebo or imipramine (dose range of 75–225 mg per day) for six weeks. At the end of the study, there were no significant differences between the two treatment groups. Bernstein and colleagues recently reported that the combination of imipramine and cognitive behavioral therapy (CBT) was significantly more effective than CBT alone in the treatment of school refusal in adolescents with comorbid depression and anxiety. The group treated with imipramine showed a faster treatment response in symptoms of depression and rate of return to school as compared to a placebo group.

There is a concern that tricyclic antidepressant use in children is associated with cardiac risk. There have been reports of children who suddenly died while being treated with normal dosages of desipramine.[81–84]

Given the uncertain clinical efficacy of TCAs for GAD, plus the significant side effects, particularly the cardiac risk, this class of medication is not a first choice. When these medications are used, the child or adolescent needs to have baseline vital signs including sitting and standing blood pressure with pulse, as well as a baseline EKG. Once the therapeutic dose is reached, the EKG should be repeated and a serum level should be checked. This should be repeated with each significant dose adjustment.

Serotonin reuptake inhibitors

The safety of the SSRIs recommends them as a choice, as does their notable effectiveness in treating depression, which is commonly comorbid with childhood anxiety disorders. The SSRIs have shown efficacy in the treatment of adult anxiety disorders, including GAD[85,86] and panic disorder.[87] Given the clinical similarity between these disorders and childhood anxiety disorders such as SAD and GAD, the favorable response to SSRIs provides a rationale for testing these medications in younger populations. Fluoxetine has shown some preliminary benefit in small pilot case series and one double-blind, placebo-controlled study in children and adolescents with anxiety disorders.[88–91]

Rynn et al[92] randomized (N=22) children meeting the diagnosis of GAD to receive either pill placebo or 50 mg (maximum dose) of sertraline for nine weeks. The Hamilton Anxiety Rating Scale (HAM-A) total score, its psychic and somatic factors and the two global assessments of illness Scales of Severity (CGS) and Improvement (CGI < 3), showed significant treatment differences in favor of sertraline over placebo from week four onwards (Fig. 12.1). Self-report measures reflected these results of treatment. However, in our study the remission rate was low (17%), which may

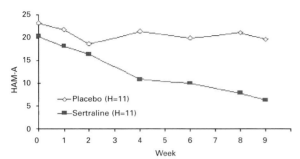

Repeated Measures ANCOVA: Treatment: $F_{(1,19)} = 18.68$; $p < 0.001$;
Time: $F_{(5,19)} = 12.74$; $p < 0.001$; Treatment by Time: $F_{(5,19)} = 6.76$; $p < 0.001$

Figure 12.1 Mean total score on the Hamilton Anxiety Rating Scale for children and adolescents with generalized anxiety disorders given sertraline or placebo in a 9-week randomized, double-blind study

be due to the short duration of treatment, the low dose (sertraline 50 mg), or the possibility that children with this illness are less likely to experience remission as compared to adults.

The Research Units of Pediatric Psychopharmacology Anxiety Study Group completed a randomized, controlled clinical trial of eight weeks of fluvoxamine (maximum dose of 300 mg) versus placebo for 128 children and adolescents with GAD, SAD, SP, and allowed for comorbid ADHD/ADD and ODD. In the fluvoxamine-treated group, 76% had a CGI < 4 as compared to the 29% in the placebo group. With these recent positive studies, it appears that SSRIs are emerging as the first line medication treatment for childhood anxiety disorders. For children with concurrent ADD/ADHD an initial trial of stimulant treatment is recommended, followed by re-evaluating the need for a trial with an antidepressant.[93,94]

There are no specific laboratory tests required for the prescribing of SSRIs. One particular concern for the prescribing clinician is the risk of drug-drug interactions. The SSRIs inhibit specific isoenzymes in the P450

cytochrome system (2D6, 1A2, 2C, and 3A4), and this is different for each medication.[95] It is important for the clinician to obtain a detailed medication history, including over-the-counter medications.

In prescribing SSRIs, it is recommended to initiate the medication at a low dose, for example, with sertraline, 25 mg for the first 7 days, and then increase to 50 mg, increasing slowly as clinical response dictates. As can be seen from the research presented, there still remains a lack of information about the amount of these medications required by this particular anxiety disorder. Once a therapeutic dose is reached, this dose should be maintained for 6–8 weeks to assess its efficacy

There have been withdrawal symptoms reported with the discontinuation of SSRIs, including nausea, headache, dizziness, and agitation.[96] Therefore, these medications should not be abruptly discontinued. From the available evidence on the effects of medications, it appears that perhaps the SSRIs would be a first-line psychopharmacological treatment for childhood GAD, if the clinical course warranted it, given its safety and tolerability.

Psychosocial treatment

The last few years have seen a rapid increase in the development and established efficacy of cognitive-behavioral approaches for childhood anxiety disorders. There are three published clinical trials on the treatment of childhood anxiety disorders (overanxious, separation anxious, and avoidant disorder) that have documented the efficacy of an individual cognitive-behavioral child treatment compared to wait list control.[52,97,98] While there is a relatively rich behavioral and cognitive-behavioral literature on the treatment of specific childhood phobias or circumscribed fears (e.g. fear of the dark, medical or dental procedures), the empirical work on treatments for the childhood non-phobic anxiety disorders is limited.[99,100] There are two published clinical trials on the treatment of childhood anxiety disorders (overanxious, separation anxious, and avoidant disorder) that have documented the efficacy of an individual cognitive-behavioral child treatment compared to wait list control.[52,98] There is some preliminary efficacy data available on a cognitive-behavioral treatment approach for childhood obsessive-compulsive disorder[101] and group-cognitive behavioral treatment for adolescents with social phobia.[102] At this time there does not appear to be any empirical dat` assessing the efficacy of other individual or family-based treatments for childhood anxiety disorders, with the exception of combined psychosocial treatment by Barrett, Dadds, and Rapee.[97] Kendall's CBT treatment approach[103] is 16 sessions long and incorporates both skill building (relaxation, modifying self-talk, problem solving, and self-reinforcement) and practice of these skills in imagined and in-vivo anxiety-provoking situations. For descriptions of the approach, see Kendall;[52] Kendall et al;[104] Kendall et al.[103] Sixty four percent[52] and 53%[98] of the children treated with CBT did not meet criteria for an anxiety diagnosis at the end of treatment. The majority of children demonstrated clinically as well as statistically significant change of anxiety and depressive symptoms, and coping skills on self-report measures at both the end of treatment and at follow-up were improved.[52,98,105] Similar results were reported by Barrett et al[97] using a modification of the Kendall Coping Cat manual. In addition, Silverman et al.[106] found that either of the two components of most CBT programs for anxiety disorders: self-control (modifying and improving self-regulation skills) or contingency management approaches (using contracts, reinforcement,

and extinction) was effective alone in the treatment of child phobic disorders.

A number of recent studies have also documented success rates for a group version of cognitive-behavioral treatment for childhood anxiety disorders that is close to or equivalent to an individual treatment format.[106–109] Albano[102] has also tested a group cognitive-behavioral treatment for adolescents with social phobia.

Parental and family involvement

Investigators have begun the empirical testing of the benefit of adding family anxiety management approaches to child-focused CBT anxiety treatment. Barrett et al.[97] compared the Kendall et al.[103] individual CBT treatment with CBT plus a behavioral family intervention (CBT-FAM). The family intervention included teaching parents: to reward courageous and coping behavior and to extinguish excessive anxious behavior; to manage their own anxiety with similar CBT techniques; and to develop new family communication and problem-solving skills. At the end of treatment, 84% of children in combined treatment no longer met DSM-IIIR diagnosis compared to 57% of children treated with CBT alone. The combined treatment continued to show superior outcome at 6-month (84% vs 71%) and 12-month follow-up (96% vs 70%). CBT-FAM also showed benefits for family-related measures (parenting competence and family disruption) and superiority on both family measures and ratings of overall anxiety, overall functioning, and avoidant behavior at follow-up. The combined treatment was especially effective for female and younger children. Barrett[107] reported close to equivalent results with group formats of these treatments as found in individual treatment.

Mendlowitz et al[110] compared child only, parent only, and child-parent groups for children with anxiety disorders. All groups showed improvement on anxiety and depressive symptoms with no difference between groups, but children in the child-parent groups used more active coping strategies post treatment than children in the other two treatment groups. Cobham et al.[108] helped clarify the benefits and limitations of the combined family treatments based on parental anxiety. They tested group treatments of the individual child CBT and one component of the family treatment package, parent anxiety management. These investigators found that children whose parents did not have anxiety did equally well in the CBT treatment only group as in a combined CBT-parent anxiety management treatment, while children whose parents did have anxiety did poorly in the child CBT treatment and did well in the combined treatment.

It is clear that parental involvement can significantly increase treatment efficacy, especially if parents have significant anxiety symptoms themselves. The CBT and family-based treatments have been tested in childhood GAD, social phobia, and avoidant disorder. The combination of teaching children skills to manage their anxiety as well as teaching parents how to interact with and help their child cope rather than allow avoidance is crucial for successful treatment in many cases.

Future directions

In terms of diagnostic issues, there is a great deal of overlap in childhood anxiety disorders and they all seem to respond to the same treatments. Could this possibly suggest that these DSM-IV anxiety diagnoses are artifacts of the present diagnostic system and may in fact be part of the same anxiety disorder?

As described in this chapter, there is strong evidence to support the effectiveness of antidepressant and cognitive-behavioral treatments for childhood GAD with or without additional comorbid anxiety disorders (SAD/SP). However, how does the clinician decide which type of treatment to initiate first? Often, this may be determined by the clinician's particular expertise, which may be pharmacotherapy, CBT, or family therapy. It appears reasonable to consider a psychosocial intervention first, providing the expertise is available in cognitive-behavioral therapy with parent training or family therapy. This treatment approach should be tried for approximately four months. If the child were not then showing a 50% reduction in anxiety symptoms, it would be reasonable to consider a medication consultation with a child psychiatrist. It remains difficult to predict which children are most likely to require medication treatment. There is no data available to shed light on the question of whether or not the sequencing of therapies or combinations of therapies leads to a difference in treatment outcome. The duration and intensity of treatment required to lead to illness remission is also not known. In particular, for treatment with antidepressants it is not known what is the appropriate maintenance therapy. The studies completed at this time are all short-term treatment studies. The National Institutes of Mental Health are funding a multi-site study, "Child/Adolescent Anxiety Multimodal Treatment Study", to address some of these issues. This is a randomized controlled trial to replicate and extend the initial findings from the psychopharmacology and CBT literatures. The first part of the study is a 12-week randomized controlled efficacy study comparing fluvoxamine, CBT, and their combination, with pill placebo in children aged 7 to 16 years with primary diagnoses of DSM-IV SAD, SP, and GAD. The second part of the study involves a 6-month treatment maintenance period for children who respond to the three active treatments. The completion of this study will hopefully provide more information to assist all of us to provide the best treatment for children who suffer from these disorders.

References

1. Kendall PC, Warman MJ, Anxiety disorders in youth: Diagnostic consistency across DSM-IIIR and DSM-IV, *J Anxiety Disord* (1996) 10:452–63.

2. Feehan M, McGee R, Raja R, Williams S, DSM-IIIR disorders in New Zealand 18 year olds, *Aust N Z J Psychiatry* (1994) 28:87–99.

3. Lewinsohn PM, Hops H, Roberts RE, Seeley JR, Andrews JA, Adolescent psychopathology: I. Prevalence and incidence of depression and other DSM-IIIR disorders in high school students, *J Abnorm Psychol* (1993) 102:133–44.

4. McGee R, Feehan M, Williams S, Partridge F, DSM-III disorders in a large sample of adolescents, *J Am Acad Child Adolesc Psychiatry* (1990) 29:611–19.

5. Anderson JC, Williams S, McGee R, Silva PA, DSM-III disorders in preadolescent children: prevalence in a large sample from the general population, *Arch Gen Psychiatry* (1987) 44:69–76.

6. Bowen RC, Offord DR, Boyle MH, The prevalence of overanxious disorder and separation anxiety disorder: results from the Ontario child health study, *J Am Acad Child Adolesc Psychiatry* (1990) 29:753–8.

7. Costello EJ, Child psychiatric disorders and their correlates: A primary care pediatric sample, *J Am Acad Child Adolesc Psychiatry* (1989) 28:851–5.

8. Kashani JH, Orvaschel H, Anxiety disorders in mid-adolescence: A community sample, *Am J Psychiatry* (1988) 145:960–4.

9. Orvaschel H, Weissman M, Epidemiology of anxiety in children. In: *Anxiety Disorders of Childhood.* Gittelman R (ed.) (New York: Guilford Press, 1986).

10. Werry J, Diagnosis and assessment. In: *Anxiety Disorders of Childhood.* Gittelman R (ed.) (New York: Guilford Press, 1986).

11. Keller MB, Lavori PW, Wunder J, Beardslee WR, Schwartz CE, Roth J, Chronic course of anxiety disorders in children and adolescents, *J Am Acad Child Adolesc Psychiatry* (1992) 31:595–9.

12. Strauss CC, Behavioral assessment and treatment of overanxious disorder in children and adolescents, *Behav Modif* (1988) 12:234–51.

13. Strauss CG, Lease CA, Kazdin AE, Dulcan M, Last C, Multi-method assessment of the social competence of anxiety disordered children, *Journal of Consulting and Clinical Psychology* (1989) 18:184–90.

14. Dweck C, Wortman C, Learned helplessness, anxiety and achievement. In *Achievement, Stress and Anxiety*, Ed HH Krone, L Laux, (New York: Hemisphere, 1982).

15. Livingston R, Taylor JL, Crawford SL, A study of somatic complaints and psychiatric diagnosis in children, *J Am Acad Child Adolesc Psychiatry* (1988) 27:185–7.

16. Kearney CA, Albano AM, *Therapist's manual for the prescriptive treatment of school refusal in youth.* (New York: Psychological Corporation, 2000).

17. Rutter M, Giller H, *Juvenile Delinquency: Trends and Perspectives* (New York: Guilford 1984).

18. Hibbett A, Fogelman K, Future lives of truants: Family formation and health-related behaviour. *British Journal of Educational Psychology,* (1990) 60:171–9.

19. Flakierskia-Praquin N, Lindtrom M, Gillberg C, School phobia with separation anxiety disorder: a comparative 20- to 29-year follow-up study of 35 school refusers. *Compr Psychiatry,* (1997) 38:17–22.

20. King NJ, Bernstein GA, School refusal in children and adolescents: a review of the past 10 years, *J Am Acad Child Adolesc Psychiatry,* (2001) 40:197–205.

21. Beidel DC, Fink CM, Turner SM, Stability of anxious symptomatology in children, *Journal of Abnormal Child Psychology* (1996) 24(3):257–68.

22. Cantwell DP, Baker L, Stability and natural history of DSM-III childhood diagnoses, *Annual Progress in Child Psychiatry and Child Development* (1989) 28(5): 311–22.

23. Dadds MR, Spence SH, Holland DE, Barrett PM, Laurens KR, Prevention and early intervention for

anxiety disorders: A controlled trial *Journal of Consulting and Clinical Psychology* (1997) 65(4):627–35.

24. Last CG, Hersen M, Kazdin AE, Finkelstein R, Strauss CC, Comparison of DSM-III separation anxiety and overanxious disorders: Demographic characteristics and patterns of comorbidity, *J Am Acad Child Adolesc Psychiatry* (1987a) 26:527–31.

25. Last CG, Perrin S, Hersen M, Kazdin AE, A prospective study of childhood anxiety disorders. *J Am Acad Child Adolesc Psychiatry* (1996) **35**: 1502-10.

26. Aronson TA, Logue CM, On the longitudinal course of panic disorder: Developmental history and predictors of phobic complications, *Comprehensive Psychiatry* (1987) 28:344–55.

27. Last CG, Strauss CC, Hersen M, Francis G, Grubb HJ, Psychiatric illness in the mothers of anxious children, *Am J Psychiatry* (1987) 144:1580–3.

28. Last CG, Phillips JE, Statfeld A, Childhood anxiety disorders in mothers and their children, *Child Psychiatry and Human Development* (1987) 18:103–12.

29. Last CG, Hansen C, Franco N, Cognitive-behavioral treatment of school phobia, *J Am Acad Child Adolesc Psychiatry* (1998) 37:404–11.

30. Andrews G, Stewart G, Allen R, Henderson AS, The genetics of six neurotic disorders: a twin study, *J Affect Disord* (1990) 19:23–9.

31. Fyer AJ, Mannuza S, Chapman TF, Liebowitz MR, Klein DF, A direct interview family study of social phobia. *Arch Gen Psychiatry* (1993) **50**:286–93.

32. Kendler K, Neale M, Kessler R, Heath A, Eaves L, The genetic epidemiology of phobias in women, *Arch General Psychiatry,* (1992) 49:273–81.

33. Torgersen S, Genetic factors in anxiety disorders, *Arch General Psychiatry* (1983) 40:1065–9.

34. Sylvester C, Hyde TS, Reichler RJ, The diagnostic interview for children in studies at risk for anxiety disorders or depression, *J Am Acad Child Adolesc Psychiatry* (1987) 26:668–75.

35. Turner SM, Beidel DC, Costello A, Psychopathology in the offspring of anxiety disorders patients, *Journal of Consulting and Clinical Psychology* (1987) 55:229–35.

36. Beidel DC, Turner SM, At risk for anxiety: I. Psychopathology in the offspring of anxious parents, *J Am Acad Child Adolesc Psychiatry* (1997) 36(7): 918–24.

37. Weissman MM, Leckman JF, Merikangas KR, Gammon GD, Prusoff BA, Depression and anxiety disorders in parents and children, *Arch Gen Psych* (1984) 41:845–52.

38. Silverman WK, Nelles WB, The anxiety disorders interview schedule for children, *J Am Acad Child Adolesc Psychiatry* (1988) 27:772–8.

39. Brady EU, Kendall PC, Comorbidity of anxiety and depression in children and adolescents, *Psychological Bulletin* (1992) 111:244–55.

40. Kovacs M, Gastonis C, Paulauskas SL, Richards C, Depressive disorders in childhood: A longitudinal study of comorbidity with and risk for anxiety disorders, *Arch Gen Psychiatry* (1989) 46:776–82.

41. Kendall PC, MacDonald J, Henin A, Treadwell K, *Parent ratings of anxiety in children: Development and validation of the CBCL-A,* Manuscript submitted for publication, Temple University, 1997.

42. Gullone E, King NJ, The fears of youth in the 1990s: Contemporary normative data, *J Genet Psychol* (1993) 154:137–53.

43. Dong Q, Yang B, Ollendick TH, Fears in Chinese children and adolescents and their relations to anxiety and depression, *J Child Psychol Psyc,* (1994) 35:351–63.

44. Fonseca A, Yule W, Erol N, Cross-cultural issues. In T. Ollendick, N. King, & W. Yule (Eds.), *International handbook of phobic and anxiety disorders in children and adolescents* New York: Plenum Press. (1994) 67–86.

45. King NJ, Gullone E, Ollendick TH, Manifest anxiety and fearfulness in children and adolescents, *J Genet Psychol* (1992) 153:63–73.

46. Schniering CA, Hudson JL, Rapee RM, Issues in the diagnosis and assessment of anxiety disorders in children and adolescents, *Clin Psychol Rev* (2000) 20:453–78.

47. March J, Albano AM, New developments in assessing pediatric anxiety disorders, *Advances in Clinical Child Psychology*, Vol. 20, eds. Thomas H Ollendick and Ronald J Prinz (New York: Plenum Press, 1998).

48. Albano AM, Silverman WK, *Anxiety Disorder Interview Schedule for DSM-IV: Child version.* (Psychological Corporation, 1996).

49. Silverman WK, Eisen AR, Age differences in the reliability of parent and child reports of child anxious symptomatology using a structured interview, *J Am Acad Child Adolesc Psychiatry* (1992) 31:117–24.

50. Silverman WK, Rabian B, Test-retest reliability of DSM-IIIR childhood anxiety disorders and symptoms using the Anxiety Disorders Interview

Schedule for Children, *J Anxiety Disorders,* (1995) 9(2):139–50.

51. Rapee RM, Barrett PM, Dadds MR, Evans L, Reliability of the DSM-IIIR childhood anxiety disorders using structural interview: Interrator and parent-child agreement, *J Am Acad Child Adolesc Psychiatry* (1994) **33**:984–92.

52. Kendall PC, Treating anxiety disorders in children: Results of a randomized clinical trial, *J Consulting and Clin Psychology,* (1994) **62**(1):100–10.

53. March J, Parker J, Sullivan K, Stallings S, Conners CK, The Multidimensional Anxiety Scale for Children (MASC): Factor structure, reliability and validity, *J Am Acad Child Adolesc Psychiatry,* (1997) **36**(4):554–65.

54. Reynolds CR, Richmond BO, What I think and feel: A revised measure of children's manifest anxiety, *Journal of Abnormal Child Psychology* (1978) 6:271–80.

55. Achenbach T, *Manual for the child behavior checklist/ 4-18 and 1991 profile* (Burlington, VT: University of Vermont, Department of Psychiatry, 1991).

56. Achenbach TM, Edelbrock CS, *Manual for the child behavior checklist and profile* (Burlington, VT: University of Vermont, 1983).

57. Gould RA, Buckminster S, Pollack MH, Otto MW, Yap L, Cognitive-behavioral and pharmacological treatment for social phobia: A meta-analysis, *Clinical Psychology: Science and Practice,* (1997) 4:291–306.

58. Gould RA, Otto MW, Pollack MP, Yap L, Cognitive-behavioral and pharmacological treatment of generalized anxiety disorder: A preliminary meta-analysis, *Behavior Therapy,* (1997) 28:285–305.

59. Brawman-Mintzer O, Lydiard RB, Biological basis of generalized anxiety disorder, *J Clin Psychiatry* (1997) **58** (suppl 3):16–25.

60. Greenblatt DJ, Shader RI, Drug Therapy. Current status of benzodiazepines: part I. *New Eng J Med* (1983) 309:354–8.

61. Rickels K, Benzodiazepines in the treatment of anxiety: North American Experiences. In: *The Benzodiazepines: From Molecular Biology to Clinical Practice.* E. Costa, ed. New York: Raven Press (1983) 295–310.

62. Rickels K, Schweizer E, Case WG, Greenblatt DJ, Long-term therapeutic use of benzodiazepines. I. effects of abrupt discontinuation, *Arch Gen Psychiatry,* (1990) 47: 899–907.

63. Graae F, Milner J, Rizzotto L, Klein RG, Clonazepam in childhood anxiety disorders, *J Am Acad Child Adolesc Psychiatry* (1994) **33**:372–6.

64. Simeon JG, Ferguson HB, Knott V, Clinical, cognitive and neurophysiological effects of alprazolam in children and adolescents with overanxious and avoidant disorders, *J Am Acad Child Adolesc Psychiatry* (1992) **31**:29–33

65. Bernstein GA, Garfinkel BD, Borchardt CM, Comparative studies of pharmacotherapy for school refusal, *J Am Acad Child Adolesc Psychiatry* (1990) **29**:773–81.

66. Kutcher SP, Mackenzie S, Successful clonazepam treatment of adolescents with panic disorder (letter to the editor). *J Clin Psychopharmacol* (1988) 8:299–301.

67. Biederman J, Clonazepam in the treatment of prepubertal children with panic-like symptoms, *J Clin Psychiatry* (1987) **48**:38–41.

68. Rickels K, Case WG, Schweizer E, Garcia-Espana F, Fridman R, Long-term benzodiazepine users: 3 years after participation in a discontinuation program, *Am J Psychiatry* (1991) **148**:757–61.

69. Coffey BJ, Review and update: Benzodiazepines in childhood and adolescence, *Psychiatr Ann* (1993) **23**:332–9.

70. Kutcher SP, Reiter S, Gardener DM et al, The pharmacotherapy of anxiety disorders in children and adolescents, *Psychiatr Clin North Am* (1992) **15**:41–66.

71. Velosa JF, Riddle, MA, Pharmacologic treatment of anxiety disorders. In: Lewis, M, Martin A, Scahill L, eds. *Child and Adolescent Psychiatric Clinics of North America: Psychopharmacology.* Philadelphia: W.B. Saunders Company (2000) 9: 119–33.

72. Pohl R, Balon R, Yergani VK, Gershon S, Serotonergic anxiolytics in the treatment of panic disorder: A controlled study with buspirone, *Psychopathology,* (1989) 22: 60–67.

73. Sheehan DV, Raj AB, Sheehan KH, Soto S, Is buspirone effective for panic disorder, *Journal of Clinical Psychopharmacology* (1990) **10**(1):3–11.

74. Simeon JG, Knott VJ, Dubois C et al, Buspirone therapy of mixed anxiety disorders in childhood and adolescence: A pilot study, *J Child Adolesc Psychopharmacol* (1994) 4:159–70.

75. Riddle MA, Bernstein GA, Cook EH, Leonard HL, March JS, Swanson JM, Anxiolytics, adrenergic agents, and naltrexone, *J Am Acad Child Adolesc Psychiatry* (1999) **38**:546–56.

76. Werry JS, Aman MG (Eds) *Practitioner's Guide to Psychoactive Drugs for Children and Adolescents.* New York: Plenum Press (1999)

77. Werry JS, Aman MG, Anxiolytics, sedatives, and miscellaneous drugs. In Werry JS, Aman MG (eds): Practitioner's Guide to Psychoactive Drugs for Children and Adolescents, ed 2. New York, Plenum Medical Book Company, (1993) 391–415.

78. Berney T, Kolvin I, Bhate SR, et al, School phobia: a therapeutic trial with clomipramine and short-term outcome, *Br J Psychiatry* (1981) 138:110–18.

79. Gittleman-Klein R, Klein DF, School phobia: diagnostic considerations in the light of imipramine effects, *J Nerv Ment Dis* (1973) 156:199–215.

80. Klein DF, Mannuzza S, Chapman T, Fyer AJ, Child panic revisited, *J Am Acad Child Adolesc Psychiatry* (1992) 31:112–6.

81. Popper CW, Ziminitzky B, Sudden death putatively related to desipramine treatment in youth: A fifth case and a review of speculative mechanisms, *J Child Adolesc Psychopharmacol* (1995) 5:283–300.

82. Riddle MA, Nelson JC, Kleinman CS et al, Case study: Sudden death in children receiving Norpramine: A review of three reported cases and commentary, *J Am Acad Child Adolesc Psychiatry* (1991) 30:104–8.

83. Riddle MA, Geller B, Ryan N: Case study, Another sudden death with a child treated with desipramine, *J Am Acad Child Adolesc Psychiatry* (1993) 32:792–7.

84. Varley CK, McClellan J, Case study: Two additional sudden deaths with tricyclic antidepressants, *J Am Acad Child Psy*, (1997) 36:390–4.

85. Pollack MH, Zaninelli R, Goddard A, McCafferty JP, Bellew KM, Burnham DB, Iyengar MK, Paroxetine in the treatment of generalized anxiety disorder: Results of a placebo-controlled, flexible-dosage trial, *J Clin Psychiatry* (2001) 62(5):350–7.

86. Rickels K, Pollack MH, Sheehan DV, Haskins JT, Efficacy of venlafaxine extended-release (XR) capsules in nondepressed outpatients with Generalized Anxiety Disorder, *Am J Psychiatry* (2000) 157:968–74.

87. Pohl RB, Wolkow RM, Clary CM, Sertraline in the treatment of panic disorder: a double-blind multi-center trial, *Am J Psychiatry* (1998) 155:1189–95.

88. Birmaher B, Waterman GS, Ryan N, et al, Fluoxetine for childhood anxiety disorders, *J Am Acad Child Adolesc Psychiatry* (1994) 33:993–9.

89. Manassis K, Bradley S, Fluoxetine in anxiety disorders, *J Am Acad Child Adolesc Psychiatry* (1994) 33:761.

90. Black B, Uhde TW, Treatment of elective mutism with fluoxetine: a double-blind placebo-controlled study, *J Am Acad Child Adolesc Psychiatry* (1994) 36:545–53.

91. Fairbanks JM, Pine DS, Tancer NK, Dummit ES, Kentgen LM, Martin J, Asche BK, Klein RG, Open fluoxetine treatment of mixed anxiety disorders in children and adolescents, *J Child and Adolesc Psychopharmacol* (1997) 7:17–29.

92. Rynn MA, Siqueland L, Rickels K, Placebo-controlled trial of sertraline in the treatment of children with generalized anxiety disorder, *Am J Psychiatry* (2001) 158(12):2008–14.

93. Pliszka SR, Greenhill LL, Crimson ML, Sedillo A, Carlson C, Conners CK, McCracken JT, Swanson JM, Hughes CW, Llana ME, Lopez M, Toprac MG, The Texans Consensus Conference Panel on Medication Treatment of Childhood Attention-Deficit/Hyperactivity Disorder: The Texas Children's Medication Algorithm Project: Report of the Texans Consensus Conference Panel on Medication Treatment of Childhood Attention-Deficit/Hyperactivity Disorder. Part I. *J Am Acad Child Adolesc Psychiatry* (2000) 39(7):908–19.

94. MTA Cooperative Group, Moderators and mediators of treatment response for children with attention-deficit/hyperactivity disorder: the Multimodal Treatment Study of Children with Attention-Deficit/Hyperactivity Disorder, *Arch Gen Psychiatry* (1999) 56:1088–96.

95. Leonard HL, March J, Rickler KC et al, Pharmacology of the selective serotonin reuptake inhibitors in children and adolescents, *J Am Acad Child Adolesc Psychiatry* (1997) 36:725–36.

96. Labellarte MJ, Walkup JT, Riddle MA, The new antidepressants. Selective serotonin reuptake inhibitors, *Pediatr Clin North Am* (1998) 45:1137–55.

97. Barrett PM, Dadds MR, Rapee RM, Family treatment of childhood anxiety: A controlled trial, *J Consult Clin Psychol* (1996) 64:333–42.

98. Kendall PC, Flannery-Schroeder E, Panichelli-Mindel SM, Southam-Gerow M, Henin A, Warman M, Therapy for youths with anxiety disorders: a second randomized clinical trial, *J Consult Clin Psychol* (1997) 65:366–80.

99. Strauss CC, Behavioral assessment and treatment of overanxious disorder in children and adolescents, *Behav Modif* (1988) 12:234–51.

100. Thyer BA, Diagnosis and treatment of child and adolescent anxiety disorders, *Behav Modif* (1991) 15:310–25.

101. March JS, Mulle K, Herbel B, Behavioral psychotherapy for children and adolescents with obsessive compulsive disorder: An open trial of a new protocol driven treatment package, *J Am Acad Child Adolesc Psychiatry* (1994) 33:333–41.

102. Albano AM, Treatment of social anxiety in adolescents, *Cognitive and Behavioral Practice* (1995) 2:271–98.

103. Kendall PC, Kane M, Howard B, Siqueland L, *Cognitive-behavioral therapy for anxious children: Treatment manual* - Revision and copyright (1989) First version Kendall, Kane and Siqueland, 1987.

104. Kendall PC, Chansky TE, Kane MT, Kim RS, Kortlander E, Ronan KR, Sessa FM, Siqueland L, *Anxiety Disorders in Youth: Cognitive-Behavioral Interventions.* New York: Macmillan Publishing (1992)

105. Kendall PC, Southam-Gerow M, Long term follow-up of a cognitive-behavioral treatment for anxiety-disorder youth, J *Consult Clin Psychol* (1996) 64:724–30.

106. Silverman WK, Kurtines WM, Ginsburg GS, Weems CF, Lumpkin P, White C, Hicks D, Treating anxiety disorders in children with group cognitive-behavioral therapy: A randomized clinical trial, *J Consult Clin Psychol* (1999) 67: 995–1003.

107. Barrett PM. Evaluation of cognitive-behavioral group treatments for childhood anxiety disorders, *J Clin Child Psychol* (1998) 27:459–68.

108. Cobham VE, Dadda MR, Spence SH, The role of parental anxiety in the treatment of childhood anxiety, *J Consult Clin Psychol* (1998) 66:893–905.

109. Flannery-Schroeder E, Kendall PC, Group and individual cognitive-behavioral treatments for youth with anxiety disorders: A randomized clinical trial, *Cognitive Ther Res* (2000) 24:251–78.

110. Mendlowitz SL, Manassis K, Bradley S, Scaptillato D, Miezitis S, Shaw BF, Cognitive-behavioral group treatments I childhood anxiety disorders: The role of parental involvement, *J Am Acad Ch Adolesc Psychiatry* (1999) 38:1223–9.

13

Generalized Anxiety Disorder in Later Life

Melinda A Stanley

Introduction

Given what is known about the prevalence and impact of generalized anxiety disorder (GAD) in younger adults (see other chapters in this volume), it should come as no surprise that GAD in later life also poses a potentially serious public health problem. Only recently, however, has a small body of literature emerged to address more directly the nature, consequences, and treatment of anxiety among older individuals. The bulk of this research has focused on identifying areas of overlap and divergence among older and younger adults with GAD, often using the growing literature from younger adults as a base upon which to build. This chapter will review the available literature in this area, with attention to the epidemiology, phenomenology, assessment, and treatment of GAD in later life.

Epidemiology

Prevalence

Community surveys report six-month prevalence rates for GAD among older adults ranging from 1.9%[1] to 7.3%.[2] This wide range is likely due to methodological variations in definitions of GAD, measures of recency, sampling strategies, and assessment tools (e.g., self-report vs. clinical ratings). The lowest figures probably seriously underestimate prevalence given the associated use of hierarchical rules disallowing the diagnosis of GAD when common co-occurring disorders (e.g., major depression, panic disorder) were present. Some data also suggest that rates of anxiety symptoms and syndromes are higher among institutionalized and homebound elderly,[3,4] although figures appear more equal when variables related to physical health status are controlled.[4]

Because most older people with anxiety or other mental health difficulties usually present for care in medical settings,[1] the prevalence of late-life GAD in these settings is a relevant issue. It is well known that the prevalence of anxiety among younger medical patients is quite high, although up to 50% of these individuals go unrecognized and untreated.[5] Recognition of anxiety in older adults is likely to be even more difficult given general tendencies among individuals in this age group to present with somatic rather than psychological symptoms.[6] The presence of increasingly frequent medical illnesses in later life also creates more complicated differential diagnostic issues that may contribute to poor recognition of anxiety and other mental health problems.[7] Recognition of GAD may be most problematic in this regard given that the core features of this disorder are more general and pervasive than is the case for other anxiety disorders. Again, however, prevalence rates for GAD in older medical patients range dramatically, from 0.8% in a general medical sample[8] to 9% among patients presenting to a specialty dizziness clinic.[9] Data from the National Ambulatory Medical Care Survey (NAMCS) suggest that anxiety disorders were diagnosed during only 1.3% of doctor's office visits made by older adults in the US in 1997, and only 11% of these individuals were assigned a diagnosis of GAD.[10] It is as yet unclear, however, whether these relatively low figures reflect true prevalence or difficulties with symptom presentation or recognition.

Impact

As noted elsewhere in this volume, GAD alone is a pervasive and chronic disorder that creates significant interference in life function. Decreased quality of life has been associated with GAD in older adults,[11] and anxiety symptoms and disorders in this age group are generally associated with decreased physical activity, poorer self-perceptions of health,

decreased life satisfaction, and increased loneliness.[12] These relationships are maintained even when data are adjusted for demographic variables, severity of chronic disease, and functional limitations. Moreover, as also is the case for younger adults, coexistent disorders are prevalent in late-life GAD. Among older adults, 48–64% of patients with GAD have at least one coexistent diagnosis.[13–15] As in the younger adult literature, other anxiety and affective disorders are the most common co-occurring syndromes, but the potential for concurrent sleep disturbance and increased alcohol use is also high among older individuals.[16] This preponderance of associated symptoms and disorders complicates the clinical picture and exacerbates the impact of GAD.

Preliminary data have also documented increased economic costs of anxiety in later life. In particular, NAMCS data suggested that a diagnosis of anxiety (or depression) in older medical patients was associated with increased physician time, and therefore increased cost to the medical system.[10] Other reports have documented increased service use in general for older individuals with generalized anxiety.[1] The relationship of depression to increased service utilization and cost for older medical patients is also well demonstrated, even with statistical controls for severity of medical illness.[17,18] Given the high rates of coexistent anxiety and depressive disorders in older adults,[19,20] many of these findings are also likely applicable to older medical patients with anxiety, in particular GAD.

Demographic and risk factors

Clinical samples of older adults with GAD, like their younger counterparts, are more likely to be women,[14,15] although community data have not confirmed that gender is a significant risk factor for GAD in later life.[2] Women may simply be more likely to present for treatment. Other risk factors for late-life GAD identified among community samples include functional limitations, poorer self-perceptions of health, lower education level, experience of extreme stress during World War II, and loneliness.[2] Preliminary data have also suggested possible ethnic differences in the prevalence of late-life GAD,[1] with the highest rates among older African-American women (3.7%), followed by non-black women (2.7%), non-black men (0.7%), and African-American men (0.3%).[4] This issue deserves further study as most surveys have failed to sample ethnic minority populations adequately.

Based on retrospective self-report, the onset of GAD appears to have a bimodal distribution in both community[1] and clinical samples.[21] A high percentage of individuals report long-term, sometimes lifelong, symptoms, while another significant percentage report more recent onset. In the latter cases, the possibility of onset following stressful life events seems reasonable.[22] However, initial data suggest few meaningful differences in clinical features as a function of self-reported age of onset.[21]

Summary

Despite some inconsistencies in available data, GAD appears to be a prevalent problem in later life, with significant impact on personal distress and functioning as well as economic correlates for both patients and the systems in which they are treated. Some risk factors have been identified, although prospective data are needed to solidify knowledge about the development, and potential prevention, of late-life GAD. More data are also needed to examine directly prevalence and recognition rates for GAD and other anxiety disorders in older medical patients.

Phenomenology

Nature of GAD

Of critical importance to meaningful advances in the field is information about the nature of GAD in older adults. In particular, future advances in prevention and treatment may depend at least partially on identification of the ways in which symptoms of late-life GAD overlap and diverge from those reported in younger adults. At present, GAD is diagnosed according to the same criteria across the life-span, although some researchers (e.g., Blazer[23]) have questioned this practice. Given current use of the same diagnostic criteria across the lifespan, however, it is not surprising to find similarities in clinical features across age groups. In one early study designed to address this issue, older adults with GAD reported elevated worry, anxiety, social fears, and depression relative to community control participants with no psychiatric diagnoses.[21] Mean scores in the GAD group were comparable to those from younger GAD samples. In a separate study, older adults with GAD also reported decreased quality of life relative to age-matched control participants. Again, means were similar to those reported in younger adults with anxiety disorders.[11] Some differences in worry content have been reported, however, between older and younger adults. Although findings are not completely consistent across reports, community samples of older adults and those with GAD have reported more worry about health and less worry about work relative to younger samples.[24,25] These data fit developmental theories about the nature of normal fears and suggest areas of focus for the assessment and treatment of late-life GAD.

Despite some of these general findings, there is of course significant potential for individual variation in clinical presentation, as is true for patients of any age. Among older adults with GAD, for example, coexistent symptoms and diagnoses are common, and the presence and/or severity of these can influence the clinical picture. Recent data suggest that the presence of coexistent depression, in fact, increases clinician-rated severity of GAD.[26] There may be valid subtypes of GAD in later life characterized by variations in worry severity, associated clinical symptoms, personality variables, and perceived social support.[27] Additionally, variables such as perceived health and financial status appear to have an impact on the characteristics of worry in older adults.[28] Finally, cultural differences might be expected to moderate clinical symptoms and presentation. However, only one study has addressed potential ethnic variability in worry, and this comparison of older Japanese Americans (JA) and European Americans (EA) found no significant group differences in severity or content of worry.[28] The authors suggest that the unexpected null findings may have resulted from demographic characteristics and acculturation status of participants in the JA group. Nevertheless, more research is needed to address potential ethnic differences in the presentation of GAD in later life.

Overlap with depression

The overlap between anxiety and depression is well documented in older adults,[19,20] as is the case with younger individuals. In fact, screening instruments for depression have been used with some success to identify older adults with GAD and other anxiety disorders.[20] A question of particular interest in this area, however, is whether the relation of these affective states, and more generally the structure of affect, differs across age groups. Relevant data might have significant implications for assess-

ment and treatment of anxiety, in particular GAD, in later life. Initial data from community samples of adults ranging in age from 18 to 87 suggested that older adults experienced less negative affect in general, including less anxiety and depression, but also less overall positive affect relative to younger and middle-aged adults.[29] In addition, affective items assessing excitation and arousal loaded less highly on positive affect for older adults, and items addressing guilt or shame were less salient to an anxiety factor in this age group. These data suggest that the meaning of affective terms and/or the experience of affective states in general may vary qualitatively across age groups.

Other data have focused more directly on the structural relation between anxiety and depression in older adults, with tests of two popular models that posit differentiation of these affective states based on content of cognitions[30] or underlying affective states.[31] The content-specificity model posits that anxiety and depression can be differentiated on the basis of thoughts that are specific to depression (personal loss or failure, negative attitudes about the past or future) or anxiety (future-oriented thoughts focused on expected danger). The tripartite affective model proposes that anxiety and depression can be differentiated based on the relative strengths of negative affect (present in both anxiety and depression), positive affect (low only in depression), and physiological hyperarousal (present only in anxiety). These models have received substantial support among younger adults, but early attempts to verify them in community samples of older individuals have been less successful. Although data from older community samples provide evidence for the separability of anxiety and depression, correlations between measures of these constructs are higher than in younger adults, and there is less support for the unique associations between anxiety/depression and underlying affective states or cognitions.[32–34] Data to date suggest that among community samples of older adults, low positive affect appears to be less specifically associated with depression[32,34] and affective states including guilt and shame are less strongly associated with anxiety.[32] More generally, there also appear to be a potentially greater number of interrelated affective states among older adults.[32,33]

In a sample of older adults with GAD, guilt and shame again were not highly associated with anxiety in the evaluation of negative affect, and positive affect was not uniquely associated with depression.[35] Some evidence was obtained for the prediction of depression with the expected type of cognitions, but anxiety was less uniquely predicted by cognitive content. Although these data taken together suggest potential changes in the experience and structure of anxiety and depression over the lifespan, the impact of a cohort effect needs to be considered given the cross-sectional nature of studies to date. Nonetheless, available data indicate that current cohorts of older adults, both those with and those without GAD, may experience anxiety and depression differently than younger adults in comparable groups.

Summary

Recent data have begun to examine the characteristics of GAD in older adults, with early studies documenting significant overlap between clinical features of the disorder in younger and older patients. The content of worry may differ for patients in different age groups, however, and individual variability in associated symptoms or disorders and demographic characteristics may impact presentation. Additional research is needed to identify more clearly patterns of individual variation, particularly those related to cultural and ethnic variables. The overlap of anxiety disorders (GAD and others) with depression appears to be higher among older than younger adults. Perhaps more importantly, however, recent studies have suggested that the structure and experience of anxiety and depression actually may differ between older and younger adults with and without diagnoses of GAD. Although longitudinal data are needed to rule out cohort effects in these findings, the data nevertheless suggest the need for caution in extrapolating theoretical models for GAD and other anxiety disorders based on younger adult samples to older individuals.

Assessment
General issues

A number of issues specific to older individuals need to be considered in the assessment of anxiety, particularly GAD, in later life. Some of these concerns are particularly salient for GAD given that the core features of this disorder are more pervasive and less discrete than in other anxiety syndromes such as specific phobias, panic disorder, and obsessive-compulsive disorder. Probably of most importance in the assessment of late-life anxiety are the potential roles of age-related physiological changes and medical issues that impact presentation and differential diagnosis. For example, age-related changes in neuroendocrine and neurochemical functioning may underlie apparent differences in the age-related experience and/or description of affect described earlier.[36] In addition, as already noted, older adults experience more medical problems in general, and many of these overlap with and/or mimic anxiety-related symptoms (e.g., cardiovascular, endocrine, pulmonary, metabolic, and neurologic diseases), making differential diagnosis a much more complicated task.[7,23,36] Similarly, older patients tend to take more medications that can produce anxiety-related adverse effects, again complicating evaluations for anxiety. Finally, current cohorts of older individuals tend to present with more somatic symptoms, often under-reporting or denying psychological problems.[6] These issues taken together emphasize the importance of a careful medical work-up and a detailed clinical interview for the assessment of anxiety in older patients.[7,23]

Increased psychological comorbidity also complicates the assessment of GAD and other anxiety disorders in older adults. Most important here is the high degree of overlap with depression described earlier.[19,20] In some practical ways, clear differentiation of GAD and depression may be unnecessary given significant commonalities in pharmacological and psychosocial approaches used to treat both sets of symptoms (see *Treatment*). However, careful differentiation is important for accurate communication of clinical information as well as for theoretical and applied research designed to extend knowledge of these two classifications of symptoms/disorders and their etiology, presentation, and treatment. Other coexistent and/or overlapping psychological conditions, in particular other anxiety disorders, sleep disorders, substance use, and behavioral agitation in dementia, also need to be considered in the assessment and differential diagnosis of GAD in later life.

In addition to these clinical issues, a number of practical considerations need to be made when assessing older adults for GAD or any other anxiety disorder. First, consideration

should be given to the use of multimodal assessment strategies whenever possible. Although a multimodal approach is always optimal, it is particularly important in the case of older adults, whose ability to self-report symptoms in the traditional ways may be impaired due to cognitive and/or communication difficulties.[36] In these cases, simplification of language used to query patients, corroboration of information from caretakers or close relatives, and the use of behavioral observation may be particularly helpful.[37] Second, even when traditional self-report and clinician-rated measures are used, procedures should be implemented to reduce the impact of age-related changes in sensory and cognitive function. For example, more time might need to be allotted for administration of measures, font size may need to be adjusted for printed instruments, and care may need to be taken to alleviate distractions in the testing environment. Finally, in order to minimize the impact of fatigue and maximize patients' ability to attend to detailed questions, assessment appointments may need to be relatively brief and/or incorporate sufficient breaks for exercise or rest.[37]

Assessment instruments

A small body of literature has accumulated to evaluate the utility of various assessment instruments to detect anxiety in older adults. The majority of this work has focused on measures with psychometric support in younger samples, probably due to the economic advantages of this strategy and the associated ability to compare clinical features across age groups. Recent reviews of the literature suggest that adequate psychometric properties have been demonstrated for a number of measures of worry and associated clinical symptoms in community samples of older adults, older psychiatric and medical outpatients, and older adults with GAD.[16,36–38] These reviews also have indicated that a number of structured diagnostic interviews appear to function well for the diagnosis of anxiety and related disorders in later life.

Of particular interest here, however, are recent empirical studies demonstrating adequate reliability and validity for self-report and clinician-rated measures of worry, anxiety, depression, quality of life, and social support among older adults with GAD.[11,39–42] This collection of measures allows for moderate breadth of assessment for both clinical and research settings. However, samples among which these instruments typically have been used include high functioning, cognitively intact, white, well-educated, and healthy older adults. Thus, additional attention is needed to examine the utility of available measures among more representative samples of older adults who are more diverse demographically and clinically. It is likely that the measures will function less well among such samples and that modifications will be needed to meet the needs of more representative groups of older individuals.

Much less attention has been given to alternative assessment strategies for evaluating anxiety among patients with serious cognitive and communication or sensory difficulties. Already noted was the potential benefit of behavioral observation strategies, which preliminary data have suggested may be an important alternative or adjunct for the assessment of late-life anxiety.[36–38] However, only preliminary efforts have been made to identify target observable behaviors for the assessment of GAD or other anxiety disorders in older adults. When a set of these is clarified, it will be important to address the ability of behavioral observation procedures to differentiate symptoms that signal anxiety from those that are the sequelae of alternative psychological or medical problems.[36]

Likewise, psychophysiological assessment has received no attention in the older adult literature. Central to the development of evaluation strategies in this area will be consideration of changes in basal arousal and physiological responsiveness that may occur as a result of normal aging, increased medical difficulties, and/or medication use.[36] Nevertheless, psychophysiological assessment procedures may prove a highly functional alternative to traditional assessment methods for the evaluation of anxiety among more impaired older adults.

Summary

Assessment of GAD in later life is a complicated task. The symptoms of GAD are more pervasive and less discrete than in other anxiety disorders, and several issues unique to older adults make diagnosing the disorder even more difficult in this population. Key issues in this regard include age-related changes in physical functioning, differences in the experience and self-report of anxiety symptoms across age groups, and the need for revisions in assessment strategies to adjust for age-related sensory or cognitive functioning. Nonetheless, empirical literature is beginning to accumulate to document the potential utility of a moderate array of measures targeting worry and related symptoms for older patients with GAD. More work is needed, however, to evaluate the usefulness of these measures for more impaired patients, who have not typically been included in studies to date. Moreover, additional research is needed to develop alternative measures that may be most useful for patients with severe cognitive, sensory, or communication deficits.

Treatment

Only a minority of older adults with anxiety reports the use of outpatient mental health services. Instead, most older adults present for care in medical settings,[1] with the primary mode of treatment generally pharmacological. Naturalistic data show that about half of older primary care patients assigned an anxiety disorder diagnosis during an outpatient visit were prescribed anxiolytic or antidepressant medication.[10] This figure increased to 85% when both anxiety and depression were diagnosed. Recently, data from clinical trials have also begun to suggest the potential benefits of psychosocial treatment, in particular cognitive behavior therapy, for late-life GAD. Data related to both of these primary treatment modalities will be reviewed here.

Pharmacological treatment

No well-controlled clinical trials have been conducted to examine the efficacy of anti-anxiety or antidepressant medications for the treatment of late-life GAD. Although early data suggested the benefits of anti-anxiety medications for older patients with undiagnosed anxiety or anxiety-related symptoms,[43] serious methodological flaws characterized these studies. The most notable of these was the failure to define clearly the nature of anxiety in study participants.[43] Nevertheless, medications with documented efficacy in younger adults are prescribed for older patients with anxiety. Benzodiazepines are probably used most often, although clinical recommendations call for lower doses of compounds with shorter half-lives to be used over a briefer interval than might be the case for younger patients.[23,43,44] These recommendations are based on age-related differences in the pharmacokinetic properties of the medications and the increased risk of adverse effects for older individuals. Benzodiazepines can, for example, impact cognitive functioning and psychomotor performance in ways that create significant consequences for life function in older adults (e.g., decreased ability to drive, increased risk of hip fractures due to falls, significant memory problems).

Some data do suggest the possible benefits of alternative anti-anxiety medications, in particular buspirone, for the treatment of late-life anxiety.[23,43,44] Relevant data with older adults, however, come only from open clinical trials and, again, none of these directly addresses the treatment of GAD. Antidepressant medications with anxiety-reducing effects in younger patients are also recommended.[23,44] Data from older adults with depression suggest that these compounds may be useful in this age group, although clinical trials are needed to evaluate the specific effects for older patients with GAD and other anxiety disorders. Of particular concern will be the potential toxicity of tricyclics, especially related to anticholinergic complications such as constipation with volvulus and the risk of death following overdose or suicide attempts.

Psychosocial treatment

The literature addressing the impact of psychosocial treatment for late-life GAD has focused on the impact of cognitive-behavior therapy (CBT) given the documented efficacy of this approach for younger patients. Moreover, the short-term, symptom-focused approach of CBT may be particularly well suited for older adults.

Early studies in this area demonstrated the benefits of cognitive-behavioral interventions, in particular relaxation training, for anxiety in community samples of older individuals with undiagnosed anxiety symptoms (see 38 and 45 for reviews). Clinical case reports have also suggested the potential utility of CBT for older adults with anxiety disorders (again, see 38 and 45 for reviews). However, only recently have controlled clinical trials targeted patients with GAD. Interventions in these studies have involved multi-component treatment programs that parallel those in the younger adult literature, including education and awareness training, cognitive therapy, and exposure.[13-15] The potential utility of additional treatment components has also been suggested, including interoceptive exposure for patients with panic, sleep management skills training, enhancement of daily structure, and skills for managing medication withdrawal.[46] In most cases, treatment has been conducted in small groups to enhance social support and decrease projected costs of the intervention. Additionally, increased visual and written materials have been incorporated to meet the needs of older individuals with age-related limitations in sensory function and memory, and attempts have been made to present material in more concrete ways that use less psychological 'jargon' that may be unfamiliar to older adults.

In the first study of CBT for GAD in later life, the effects of CBT were compared to a nondirective supportive psychotherapy (SP) condition for 48 adults aged 55 and older.[13] Results showed significant improvements following both CBT and SP in worry, anxiety, and depression. Effect sizes were large, and gains were maintained over a 6—month follow-up interval. However, results of this initial trial were limited due to significant methodological problems, the most notable of which was the absence of an adequate control condition against which to compare the effects of either intervention. Also, patient symptoms and treatment integrity were not evaluated by independent experts, patients were younger than is typical in older adult research, and the

follow-up interval was relatively brief.

Three subsequent studies of CBT for late-life GAD, each of which addresses some of the limitations of earlier work, have now been conducted. In one trial, Wetherell and colleagues[15] compared the effects of CBT with a discussion group (DG) and a wait-list control condition (WL). CBT in this trial was comparable to the Stanley et al.[13] study, and results indicated improvements in both active treatment conditions (CBT, DG) relative to WL. Slight advantages were noted for CBT over DG in self-reported time spent worrying, depression, and quality of life. Gains were maintained or enhanced over follow-up. However, participants were relatively young (55 years or older) and the follow-up interval was only 6 months.

Results from another more recent study by the author and colleagues[14] suggested the benefits of CBT relative to a minimal contact control condition (MCC). Improvements were noted on measures of worry, anxiety, depression, specific fears, and quality of life for patients aged 60 and over. Response rates were 45% for CBT and 8% for MCC. These rates were slightly higher than in prior reports,[13,15] although all of these studies have produced lower responder rates than in the younger adult literature. Wait-list responder rates are also lower in the older adult GAD literature.[14,15] These data suggest that GAD may be more difficult to treat in older adults and may require additional intervention modifications for optimal use in this age group. It is also possible that the group format used in these studies is less efficacious than the individual treatment studied most often with younger patients.

In the Stanley et al.[14] study, improvements for patients in CBT were maintained over one-year follow-up. Exploratory predictor analyses also suggested the potential utility of pretreatment symptom severity, treatment expectancy and credibility, and generalized measures of self-efficacy and optimism for identifying improved response. These data overlap to some degree with studies of younger adults with GAD, but patterns are not consistent across the older adult literature.[15] Future research will need to address this issue with larger samples than heretofore have been available.

Preliminary results from one additional study by Gorenstein and colleagues[47] suggested the utility of CBT plus medication management (MM) relative to MM alone for older adults with GAD who were also regular users of anti-anxiety medication. Treatment in this trial was broader than in the other studies, with a wide array of components included to address not only the core cognitive and physiological symptoms of GAD, but also to target sleep difficulties, problem-solving deficits, panic symptoms, medication withdrawal, and the need for increased daily structure. Final results of this trial have not yet been reported, although the authors report that findings are in line with preliminary analyses (Gorenstein, personal communication).

These studies taken together provide exciting data regarding the potential utility of psychosocial treatments, in particular CBT, for the improvement of symptoms in older adults with GAD. All of the data are limited, however, in a number of ways. First, all outcome data to date have been collected in academic clinical settings, limiting generalizability to medical settings where older adults with anxiety typically present for care. Second, participants in all outcome studies to date have comprised homogeneous samples of older adults who are relatively young, mostly white, well educated, physically healthy, and high functioning. Third, for the most part, interventions in previous clinical trials are not well suited to more 'real world' settings given the large number of sessions required and relative lack of flexibility in the structure of treatment. A briefer and more flexible intervention may be needed to meet the individual needs of more heterogeneous and impaired patients typically seen in primary care settings. Although the Gorenstein et al.[46] treatment program incorporates increased flexibility relative to the other intervention packages studied to date, its applicability to a more heterogeneous sample of older medical patients has not been investigated.

In a very recent pilot project, the author and colleagues have begun to examine the potential utility of a revised version of CBT for late-life GAD in primary care patients.[48] Participants have been recruited from internal medicine and geriatric clinics of two large managed care organizations. Treatment includes education and awareness training, relaxation, cognitive therapy, graduated exposure, problem-solving skills training, and sleep management. The intervention is administered flexibly on an individual basis for eight sessions, with the option of two additional sessions for patients who experience crises or have difficulty learning coping skills. Preliminary data suggest the potential utility of the intervention relative to usual care (UC), but sample sizes are still very small and firm conclusions await the collection of additional data.

Summary

Late-life GAD is probably treated most often with medication. Data from younger adults suggest that anti-anxiety and/or antidepressant compounds may result in significant improvements for patients of older ages. However, recommendations regarding prescription strategies suggest that modifications need to be made in choice of medication, dosing patterns, and duration of treatment based on differences in treatment response and experience of adverse effects. Psychosocial interventions, in particular CBT, may serve as useful adjuncts or alternatives for the treatment of late-life GAD. Data from at least four clinical trials now suggest the potential efficacy of CBT in this population, although additional research is needed to examine the effectiveness of this approach in more 'real world' settings where patients are most likely to receive care. Efforts are ongoing in this area of research.

Future directions

Although GAD in older adults appears to be a relatively common and significant concern, more data are needed to address the prevalence, recognition, and impact of the disorder in medical settings where older adults most often present for care. Given the medical conditions and functional limitations experienced by patients in these settings, as well as the heterogeneity in cultural and socioeconomic variables that may impact on the experience and/or expression of anxiety, identification and diagnosis of anxiety for these patients becomes a very complicated task. However, early detection of patients appropriate for anxiety treatment is probably key to reducing the functional and economic impact of GAD in later life.

Relatedly, there is the need for increased attention to the nature and experience of anxiety for older patients. Of particular interest are the impacts of individual differences and sociocultural variables, as well as the overlap of anxiety with depression. With regard to the latter, longitudinal studies may be of most importance to test the notion that the experience of affect, in general, and the relation of anxiety and depression, more specifically, changes over the lifespan. The roles of age-related neurophysiological changes in the experience and expression of affect is also an understudied area.

Although a number of traditional self-report and clinician-rated assessment tools for evaluating anxiety appear to be useful for older adults with and without a diagnosis of GAD, little research has addressed the need for development of alternatives to assess anxiety from a broader range of perspectives (e.g., behavioral observation, psychophysiological). Likewise, little attention has been given to the development of assessment approaches uniquely suited for patients with cognitive, sensory, or communication impairments, in which cases more traditional methods may be inappropriate.

Finally, of major interest is future research on the treatment of late-life GAD. Surprisingly, very little is known about the unique impact of pharmacological interventions in older patients despite relatively large amounts of data documenting the impact of anti-anxiety and antidepressant medication in younger patients with GAD. Well-controlled trials with well-diagnosed patients are sorely needed. A growing body of literature has begun to document the utility of psychosocial interventions, in particular CBT, for late-life GAD. However, future research is needed to document the effectiveness of these approaches for a more representative group of patients seen in real-world settings.

References

1. Blazer D, George LK, Hughes D, The epidemiology of anxiety disorders: An age comparison. In: Salzman C, Lebowitz BD, eds, *Anxiety in the Elderly: Treatment and Research* (Springer Publishing Company: New York, 1991) 17–30.

2. Beekman ATF, Bremmer MA, Deeg DJH, van Balkom AJLM, Smit JH, de Beurs E, van Dyck R, & van Tilburg W, Anxiety disorders in later life: A report from the longitudinal aging study Amsterdam, *Int J Geriatr Psychiatry* (1998) 13:717–26.

3. Cheok A, Snowdon J, Miller R, Vaughan R, The prevalence of anxiety disorders in nursing homes, *Int J Geriatr Psychiatry* (1996) 11:405–10.

4. Bruce ML, McNamara R, Psychiatric status among the homebound elderly: An epidemiologic perspective, *J Am Geriatr Soc* (1992) 40:561–6.

5. Barlow DH, Lerner JA, Esler JL, Behavioral health care in primary care settings: Recognition and treatment of anxiety disorders. In: Resnick RJ, Rozensky RH, eds *Health Psychology Through the Life Span: Practice and Research Opportunities* (American Psychological Association: Washington, DC, 1996).

6. Gurian BS, Minor JH, Clinical presentation of anxiety in the elderly. In: Salzman C, Lebowitz BD, eds, *Anxiety in the Elderly: Treatment and Research* (Springer Publishing Company: New York, 1991), 21–44.

7. Kim HF, Braun U, Kunik ME, Anxiety and depression in medically ill older adults, *J Clin Geropsychology* (2001) 7:117–30.

8. Barrett JE, Barrett JA, Oxman TE, Gerber PD, The prevalence of psychiatric disorders in a primary care practice, *Arch Gen Psychiatry* (1998) 45:1100–6.

9. Sloane PD, Harman M, Mitchell CM, Psychological factors associated with chronic dizziness in patients aged 60 and older, *JAGS* (1994) 42:847–52.

10. Stanley MA, Roberts RE, Bourland SL, Novy DM, Anxiety disorders among older primary care patients, *J Clin Geropsychology* (2001) 7:105–16.

11. Bourland SL, Stanley MA, Synder AG, Novy DM, Beck JG, Averill PM, Swann AC, Quality of life in older adults with generalized anxiety, *Aging and Mental Health* (2000) 4:315–23.

12. De Beurs E, Beekman ATF, van Balkom AJLM, Deeg DJH, van Dyck R, van Tilburg W, Consequences of anxiety in older persons: Its effect on disability, well-being and use of health services, *Psychological Medicine* (1999) 29:583–93.

13. Stanley MA, Beck JG, Glassco JD, Treatment of generalized anxiety in older adults: A preliminary comparison of cognitive-behavioral and supportive approaches, *Behavior Therapy* (1996) 27:565–81.

14. Stanley MA, Beck JG, Novy DM, Averill PM, Swann AC, Diefenbach GJ, Hopko DR, Cognitive behavioral treatment of late-life generalized anxiety disorder, *Manuscript under review*.

15. Wetherell JL, Gatz M, Craske MG, Treatment of generalized anxiety disorder in older adults, *Journal of Consulting and Clinical Psychology* (in press).

16. Stanley MA, Beck JG, Anxiety disorders. In: Edelstein B, ed, *Clinical Geropsychology*, Vol. 8 in Hersen M, Bellack A, eds, *Comprehensive Clinical Psychology* (Elsevier Science Ltd., 1998), 171–91.

17. Callahan CM, Hui LL, Nienaber NA, Musick BS, Tierney WM, Longitudinal study of depression and health services use among elderly primary care patients. *J Am Geriatr Soc* (1994) 42:833–8.

18. Koenig HG, Kuchibhatla M, Use of health services by medically ill depressed elderly patients after hospital discharge, *Am J Geriatr Psychiatry* (1999) 155:871–7.

19. Beekman ATF, de Beurs E, van Balkom AJLM, Deeg DJH, van Dyck R, van Tilburg W, Anxiety and depression in later life: Co-occurrence and communality of risk factors, *Am J Psychiatry* (2000) 157:89–95.

20. Lenze EJ, Mulsant BH, Shear MK, Schulberg HC, Dew MA, Begley AE, Pollack BG, Reynolds CF, Comorbid anxiety disorders in depressed elderly patients, *Am J Psychiatry* (2000) 157:722–8.

21. Beck JG, Stanley MA, Zebb BJ, Characteristics of generalized anxiety disorder in older adults: A descriptive study, *Behav Res Ther* (1996) 34:225–34.

22. Ganzini L, McFarland BH, Cutler D, Prevalence of mental disorders after catastrophic financial loss, *J Nerv Ment Dis* (1990) 178:680–95.

23. Blazer DG, Generalized anxiety disorder and panic disorder in the elderly: A review, *Harv Rev Psychiatry* (1997) 39:18–27.

24. Diefenbach GJ, Stanley MA, Beck JG, Worry content reported by older adults with and without generalized anxiety disorder, *Aging Ment Health* (2001) 5:269–74.

25. Person DC, Borkovec TD, Anxiety disorders among the elderly: Patterns and issues, Paper presented at the 103rd annual meeting of the American Psychological Association, New York (August 1995).

26. Hopko DR, Bourland SL, Stanley MA et al., Generalized anxiety disorder in older adults: Examining the relation between clinician severity ratings and patient self-report measures, *Depress Anxiety* (2000) 12:217–25.

27. Hopko DR, Novy DM, Stanley MA et al., *An empirical taxonomy of older adults diagnosed with generalized anxiety disorder*. Poster presented at the 35th Annual Convention for the Association for Advancement of Behavior Therapy (November 2001) Philadelphia.

28. Watari KF, Brodbeck C, Culture, health, and financial appraisals: Comparison of worry in older Japanese Americans and European Americans, *J Clin Geropsychology* (2000) 6:25–39.

29. Lawton MP, Kleban MH, Dean J, Affect and age: Cross-sectional comparisons of structure and prevalence, *Psychol Aging* (1993) 8:165–75.

30. Beck AT, Brown G, Steer RA, Eidelson JI, Risking JH, Differentiating anxiety and depression: A test of the cognitive content-specificity hypothesis, *J Abnorm Psychology* (1987) 96:179–83.

31. Clark LA, Watson D, Tripartite model of anxiety and depression: Psychometric evidence and taxonomic implications, *J Abnorm Psychology* (1991) 100:316–36.

32. Shapiro AM, Roberts JE, Beck JG, Differentiating symptoms of anxiety and depression in older adults: Distinct cognitive and affective profiles, *Cognitive Therapy and Research* (1999) 23:53–74.

33. Meeks S, Woodruff-Borden J, Depp C, Structural differentiation of self-reported depression and anxiety in late life, Paper presented at the 34th annual convention for the Association for Advancement of Behavior Therapy, New Orleans (November, 2000).

34. Wetherell JL, Gatz M, Pedersen NL, A longitudinal analysis of anxiety and depressive symptoms, *Psychol Aging* (2001) 16:187–95.

35. Beck JG, Novy DM, Diefenbach GJ et al., Differentiating anxiety and depression in anxious older adults: Implications for cognitive and affective models. *Manuscript under review.*

36. Kogan JN, Edelstein BA, McKee DR, Assessment of anxiety in older adults: Current status, *J Anxiety Disord* (2000) 14:109–32.

37. Beck JG, Stanley MA, Assessment of anxiety disorders in older adults: Current concerns, future prospects. In: Antony MM, Orsillo SM, Roemer L, eds, *Practitioners' Guide to Empirically Based Measures of Anxiety*, (Kluwer Academic/Plenum Press, 2001).

38. Stanley MA, Beck JG, Anxiety disorders, *Clin Psychol Rev* (2000) 20:731–54.

39. Stanley MA, Novy DM, Bourland SL, Beck JG, Averill PM, Assessing older adults with generalized anxiety: A replication and extension, *Beh Res Ther* (2001) 39: 221–35.

40. Diefenbach GJ, Stanley MA, Beck JG, Novy DM, Averill PM, Swann AC, Examination of the Hamilton scales in assessment of anxious older adults: A replication and extension, *J Psychopathology and Behavioral Assessment* (2001) 23:117–24.

41. Snyder AG, Stanley MA, Novy DM, Averill PM, Beck JG, Measures of depression in older adults with generalized anxiety disorder: A psychometric evaluation, *Depress Anxiety* (2000) 11:114–20.

42. Stanley MA, Beck JG, Zebb BJ, Psychometric properties of the MSPSS in older adults, *Aging Ment Health* (1998) 2:186–93.

43. Salzman C, Pharmacologic treatment of the anxious elderly patient. In: Salzman C, Lebowitz B, eds, *Anxiety in the Elderly: Treatment and Research* (Springer Publishing Company: New York, 1991), 149–73.

44. Shiekh JI, Cassidy EL, Treatment of anxiety disorders in the elderly: Issues and strategies, *J Anxiety Disord* (2000) 14:173–90.

45. Wetherell JL, Treatment of anxiety in older adults, *Psychotherapy* (1998) 35:444–58.

46. Gorenstein EE, Papp LA, Kleber MS, Cognitive behavioral treatment of anxiety in later life, *Cognitive and Behavioral Practice* (1999) 6:305–20.

47. Gorenstein EE, Papp LA, Kleber MS, CBT for anxiety and anxiolytic drug dependence in later life: Interim report. In Stanley MA (chair), symposium, *Assessment and Treatment of Anxiety in Late Life, 33rd annual convention of the Association for Advancement of Behavior Therapy* (November, 1999) Toronto.

48. Stanley MA, Hopko D, Diefenbach G, Bourland S, Brothers A, Reas D, Rodriguez H, *Treating GAD in older primary care patients*. Poster presented at the 35th Annual Convention for the Association for Advancement of Behavior Therapy (November, 2001).

V   Concluding chapter

14

Generalized Anxiety Disorder: The Way Forward

Dan J Stein, Karl Rickels and David Nutt

Previous chapters in this volume have covered the phenomenology, psychobiology, pharmacotherapy, and psychotherapy of generalized anxiety disorder (GAD). In this final chapter, we review some of the central themes that have emerged, consider issues relevant to developing an algorithm for the pharmacotherapy of GAD, and outline potential avenues for future research on this disorder.

Themes in GAD

Phenomenology of GAD

We now know that GAD is an independent psychiatric disorder characterized by anxious expectation and by psychic and somatic tension that is prevalent, persistent, and disabling. Although chronic anxiety has long been recognized by clinicians, this set of important points of information about GAD has taken a while to become clarified. It is worth considering some of the conceptual and

methodological barriers that have faced clinicians and researchers, so as to ensure that recent advances are fully consolidated in the future.

The conclusion that GAD is an independent psychiatric disorder could only be made by demonstrating that the original conception of GAD as a residual diagnosis was incorrect. In his elegant chapter in this volume, Kessler persuasively marshals the evidence that defeats this early view. GAD symptoms and risk factors are specific, and pure GAD is at least as impairing as other mood and anxiety disorders. Further, although comorbidity in GAD is high, it is no higher than in depression, and it does not predict course of GAD. Unfortunately, anxiety symptoms remain more commonly disregarded by clinicians than depressive symptoms, particularly in primary care.[1]

Despite the recognition of GAD as an independent disorder, it is crucial for clinicians to be aware of comorbidity and its negative impact.[2] GAD patients should be assessed for comorbid psychiatric and medical disorders, while patients with a range of psychiatric and medical disorders should routinely be assessed for GAD. GAD in depression is associated with treatment resistance, and more attention shall be given to the impact of GAD on the onset and course of other psychiatric disorders. Also, clinicians may too easily assume that anxiety in patients with medical disorders is normal and understandable, rather than a symptom of a disorder such as GAD that may ultimately worsen the prognosis of medical comorbidity.

That patients with chronic anxiety suffer from anxious expectation and tension has been known for some time.[3] Revisions to the DSM diagnostic criteria have increasingly allowed a diagnosis that is reliable and specific (Chapter 2). Nevertheless, despite the fact that somatic symptoms are most commonly the presenting complaint of GAD patients in primary care, DSM has increasingly emphasized psychic symptoms in GAD, particularly 'excessive worry'. There is a persuasive argument that chronic worrying may not equate with severe anxiety or associated somatic symptoms, and that the criteria for GAD should focus less on worry and require more associated somatic symptoms.[4]

Furthermore, Borkovec (Chapter 8) argues that worry is best conceptualized as a secondary avoidance mechanism, in response to the primary anxiety and distinctive tension of GAD. Interestingly, older people are more likely to worry.[5] Also, determining whether worry is 'excessive' can be problematic, particularly for patients living in adverse circumstances or in patients with medical comorbidity. The dropping of the requirement of excessive worry in ICD-10 may contribute to the higher prevalence of ICD-10 GAD compared to DSM-IV GAD in community studies. In post-traumatic stress disorder, diagnostic criteria have evolved to avoid similar judgments having to be made.

The knowledge that GAD is prevalent, persistent, and disabling is increasingly supported by a range of community and clinical studies. Prevalence is particularly high in primary care settings, where GAD and depression are the most common psychiatric disorders. 'Anxiety neurosis' and subthreshold GAD have a much higher prevalence than GAD, yet are associated with significant impairment, strengthening the argument that DSM-IV criteria GAD may be overly restrictive.[6] Although there is currently relatively little cross-national data on GAD, that which does exist indicates that prevalence is roughly similar across countries.[7,8]

There is wide agreement that GAD is a persistent disorder. Although there is an increase in prevalence of GAD at around 35 to 45 years of age, with GAD the most prevalent anxiety disorder in later life, patients may demonstrate early behavioral inhibition, and spontaneous remission occurs only in a minority. Whether the diagnostic criteria for GAD should be several months (as in ICD-10) or 6 months (as in DSM-IV) is controversial. The term 'double anxiety', proposed by Rickels and Schweizer,[9] is useful in so far as it emphasizes that GAD may involve trait anxiety plus episodic anxiety.

There is also growing evidence that GAD is an impairing disorder (Chapter 2). Indeed, in a remarkable recent study of a wide range of general medical disorders, the condition associated with the highest overall dysfunction was GAD.[6] Certainly, a number of studies have suggested that associated disability is higher in GAD than in depression[10] or chronic somatic diseases.[8] In contrast to other anxiety disorders, GAD prevalence is higher in primary care than in the population; high medical utilization by GAD patients likely contributes to its costs.

Unfortunately, despite the growing awareness that GAD is an independent psychiatric disorder characterized by psychic and somatic tension that is prevalent, persistent, and disabling, people with GAD uncommonly present for treatment, and GAD is frequently underdiagnosed and undertreated. The reasons for this remain to be fully clarified (Chapters 1 and 2). It is notable, however, that in primary care practice, a psychiatric diagnosis is less likely to be given to patients with somatic presentations than to those with psychosocial complaints.[11] Furthermore, GAD patients may fail to seek help because they do not realize they have a disorder.

The discrepancy between the obvious importance of GAD and its relative neglect has clear clinical implications. First, screening questions for the presence of GAD ought to be part of every psychiatric assessment (Table 14.1). Second, screening for the presence of GAD should be a routine component of medical assessments in primary care settings, particularly in patients with unexplained somatic symptoms. Third, GAD should be considered not only in general adult practice, but also in pediatric and geriatric settings. Finally, education of consumers through the use of awareness campaigns and other interventions is crucial.

Psychobiology of GAD

Given the importance of GAD, surprisingly little is understood about its psychobiology. Nevertheless, there is a growing database pointing to the role of cognitive biases and worry processes in mediating GAD (Chapters 4 and 8), and to the involvement of specific neurotransmitter and neuroanatomical systems (Chapters 5 and 6). This knowledge helps provide a preliminary account of how specific psychotherapeutic and pharmacotherapeutic

Table 14.1 Psychiatric assessment
During the past 4 weeks, have you been bothered by feeling worried, tense, or anxious most of the time?
Are you frequently tense, irritable and having trouble sleeping?

interventions may exert their effects during the treatment of GAD.

Borkovec (Chapter 8) makes the important point that worry itself may be an avoidance mechanism. In most anxiety disorders there is primary fear and secondary avoidance. Furthermore, it seems that worrying is associated with an early decrease in somatic activation. Unfortunately, avoidant worrying may over the longer term lead to increased anxiety and worry, so resulting in a vicious cycle of symptom exacerbation. This process is arguably reminiscent of learning phenomena seen in experiments with laboratory animals (Mineka, this volume), and certainly constitutes an important target for psychotherapeutic intervention.

From a neurobiological perspective, an immediate challenge is to integrate the range of findings from animal laboratory research, pharmacological challenge studies, and functional brain imaging. It is likely that a range of neurocircuits, including amygdala circuits (involved in fear conditioning) and fronto-striatal circuits (which interact with amygdala-based circuits) play a role (Chapter 5). Genetic and environmental factors, and their complex interaction, contribute to the shaping of these neurocircuits (Chapter 6). The neurotransmitters that innervate these circuits and mediate their functioning are an important target for pharmacological treatment.

The extent to which GAD and major depression are mediated by overlapping factors remains controversial; with conflicting views, for example, about the extent to which there is an overlap in their genetic bases. The frequent temporal sequence of GAD followed by depression[12] does suggest some overlap in underlying mechanisms or risk factors. On the other hand, functional imaging shows overactivity in frontal and other regions in GAD, but decreased activity across many neurocircuits in depression (Chapter 5). Similarly, early studies suggested that different kinds of environmental stressors differentially promoted GAD and depression.[13]

Another area where much remains to be learned is that concerning the cross-cultural aspects of GAD. Presumptive variation in the experience and expression of GAD from time to time, and place to place, has not been well documented. Nevertheless, there do seem to be differences in the range of somatic symptoms across different patient populations. At the same time, symptoms of GAD, and the comorbidity of anxiety with depression and somatization, are universal phenomena.

All in all, while there have been advances in our understanding of the psychobiology of GAD, additional work is needed to delineate more precisely the pathogenesis of GAD and the mechanisms through which effective pharmacotherapy and psychotherapy act. There has been a great deal of theoretical debate about whether GAD represents a trait or a state (Chapter 4); in the future we can perhaps expect such theory to be replaced by a more integrative clinical approach (for example, emphasizing the concept of 'double anxiety') together with a detailed understanding of the psychobiological mechanisms that produce GAD symptoms.

Treatment of GAD

Fortunately, a range of safe and effective treatments for GAD is now available. These include both pharmacotherapeutic and psychotherapeutic interventions. While there is relatively little work addressing the optimal sequencing and combination of different modalities of treatment in GAD, a growing number of studies support the use of particular medications and particular psychotherapies for the management of this condition.

Sedative agents have been used for the control of anxiety throughout history. The introduction of the benzodiazepines, with their relatively safe profile in comparison to earlier barbiturates and their clear efficacy in controlled studies (particularly for somatic symptoms), was a major step forward. These agents replaced all other sedative agents for the treatment of anxiety symptoms for many years, although more recently there has been renewed interest in hydroxyzine, an antihistamine that does not have the withdrawal problems of the benzodiazepines.

The introduction of buspirone, which does not impair psychomotor function and is not associated with withdrawal problems, offered additional hope for the field. Initial clinical impressions that buspirone was not as effective as benzodiazepines were likely due to its relatively slow onset of action, and to a lack of sedation in patients inappropriately switched from benzodiazepines to buspirone (Chapter 10). Certainly, many clinical trials have found buspirone to have anxiolytic efficacy equivalent to the benzodiazepines and better than placebo.

The demonstration that antidepressants were effective not only in depression but also in GAD (particularly for psychic anxiety), overturned earlier dogma sharply differentiating the effects of benzodiazepines (on anxiety) and antidepressants (on depression). Introduction of novel antidepressants further invigorated research in this area, providing agents that are not only effective for GAD but also for a broad range of comorbid mood and anxiety disorders. Theoretically, these agents reverse both the trait and the state anxiety that characterize GAD. Furthermore, they are better tolerated than the older tricyclic antidepressants.

Psychotherapy also has a long history in the treatment of anxious patients. The most thoroughly researched psychotherapeutic intervention for GAD is cognitive-behavioral therapy (CBT). Components of CBT include self-monitoring of anxiety, relaxation training, cognitive restructuring, and imagery rehearsal. While it is currently unclear which of these components are most important, a number of rigorous and controlled studies have provided clear evidence of the overall efficacy of CBT for the treatment of GAD. These include a number of studies of late-life GAD.

One area that has not perhaps been sufficiently highlighted in the recent literature is the psychodynamics of working with GAD patients. Of particular importance is the fact that many of these patients may be perceived by clinicians as 'complainers'. Certainly, an association between high medical care utilizers described as 'frustrating patients' and GAD/somatization has been documented.[14] A supportive clinician-patient relationship is likely to be a key component of successful treatment of GAD.

In the next section, we attempt to develop an algorithm for the pharmacotherapy of adult GAD. Algorithms run the risk of oversimplifying complex medical decision-making, and certainly they cannot be applied without clinical judgment. Nevertheless, algorithms are useful in so far as they summarize the relevant considerations in medical decision-making, integrate the current empirical data, and point to gaps where future research is required.[15]

Pharmacotherapy algorithm

In considering a pharmacotherapy algorithm for adult GAD, three questions can be posed: 1) What is the first-line medication treatment for GAD?; 2) For how long should one continue such treatment for GAD?; and 3) What is the optimal pharmacotherapy of treatment-resistant patients? In this section we draw extensively on the conclusions reached in a recent GAD consensus conference in which we participated.[16]

Although this section does not consider the question of how to prioritize or combine pharmacotherapy and psychotherapy in the management of GAD, it should be emphasized that certain elements of CBT (self-monitoring diary, relaxation training, setting aside a 'worry time') are relatively easy to institute, and could be strongly considered for most GAD patients. Furthermore, a supportive clinician-patient relationship may play an important part in improving prognosis.

First-line treatment

The benzodiazepines have long been used for GAD. They are effective and are reasonably safe in the short term. Nevertheless, they are sedatives, and long-term use may be associated with increased risk of depression as well as the significant problem of potential withdrawal reactions. These agents should therefore be restricted to the short-term treatment of subthreshold GAD or an acute anxiety state, where a rapid reduction of symptoms is required. They may also be useful for intermittent or episodic use, or as adjunctive therapy during exacerbation of GAD. Particular care needs to be taken when using benzodiazepines in the elderly (Chapter 13).

Buspirone and hydroxyzine have been recommended by some authors for the treatment of GAD. Certainly these agents are safe, and there are no concerns about withdrawal reactions. Nevertheless, not all studies of buspirone in GAD are persuasive, and hydroxyzine, like the benzodiazepines, has sedative properties. Importantly, neither agent is effective for the comorbid disorders frequently found in GAD. In general, these agents should not be used as first-line interventions for GAD. Hydroxyzine may, however, have a role for the short-term treatment of acute anxiety states.

Antidepressants have increasingly been shown to be effective in the treatment of GAD. Early work demonstrated the efficacy of certain tricyclics. More recently introduced antidepressants (from the SNRI and SSRI classes) have been more vigorously studied, and have the advantage of superior tolerability. They offer a particular advantage in the long-term treatment of GAD in view of their efficacy, tolerability, and broad spectrum of actions.

Few other agents have been extensively studied in GAD. There are interesting preliminary data on pregabalin in GAD, but further work is needed before this agent can be recommended for clinical practice. Antipsychotics are prescribed by some clinicians for anxious patients, but there is currently insufficient evidence to support this practice, and these agents have clear potential for significant adverse events.[17]

In summary, we recommend SSRIs, SNRIs, and non-sedating tricyclics as the first line of treatment of adult GAD. The recent consensus conference on GAD[16] emphasized that the SSRIs and SNRIs would be particularly useful options in patients with a long-term condition, with comorbid conditions, or with suicide risk. The SSRIs are also increasingly seen as a first-line choice of medication in pediatric GAD (Chapter 12), although further trials are needed in GAD across the life cycle (Chapter 13).

Maintenance pharmacotherapy

There is a relative dearth of long-term studies of GAD. An early study found that on follow-up of patients treated with buspirone or the benzodiazepine clorazepate, buspirone was associated with fewer anxiety symptoms and a higher drop-out, perhaps suggesting that these patients relied more on their coping skills. More recent work has demonstrated in controlled studies that the effects of the SNRI venlafaxine and the SSRI paroxetine are maintained over the longer term (6 months).

On the other hand, there is good data showing that when GAD is a comorbid condition, it often precedes the development of subsequent depression or other anxiety disorders. While a range of reasons have been put forward to explain this temporal sequence, ultimately its underlying pathogenesis is not well understood. Nevertheless, many clinicians feel that early and robust treatment of GAD may well prevent comorbidity and disability.

We would suggest that the pharmacotherapy of GAD with antidepressants should be continued for at least a year. Factors that would influence a clinician to extend maintenance pharmacotherapy further include the severity of the anxiety and the history of comorbid disorders. We recognize that further studies are needed to provide empirical support for this recommendation, but in the absence of such data it would seem reasonable.

Treatment resistance

Many GAD patients fail to respond to the first medication (or psychotherapy) that is initiated. Obvious reasons for non-response should be ruled out. These include comorbidity (including comorbidity of substance use disorders and personality disorders), insufficient dose and duration of medication, and non-adherence to treatment. Nevertheless, some cases of treatment-refractory GAD will continue to be present (defined as failure to respond to two trials of adequate dose and duration).

Work on depression suggests that switching from one class of agent to another or even switching between medications from the same class, may be beneficial. To our knowledge, there are no similar studies in GAD patients. Extrapolating from clinical experience and from the depression data, however, it would seem reasonable to be hopeful that further switching of medications may be effective. Our recommendation would be to switch between different first-line agents (SSRIs, SNRIs) before attempting other agents.

There is also a lack of information about combining different medications in GAD. Of course, it would be possible to combine antidepressants with benzodiazepines or buspirone. Further work is needed, however, to demonstrate the efficacy and tolerability of such potential strategies, as well as to consider the use of agents with relatively novel mechanisms of action (e.g. pregabalin) in patients who have not benefited from standard pharmacotherapeutic interventions.

Future research

While DSM-IV criteria for GAD are a clear improvement over the DSM-III criteria, further evolution is likely to be required. Concerns about the current emphasis of DSM-IV on 'worry', for example, were emphasized earlier. Diagnostic criteria for GAD in children are also likely to require further refinement. The Hamilton Anxiety Scale remains the gold standard rating scale in GAD research; those who have worked with this instrument will be aware of the many difficulties that raters have in using it. Additional outcome measures (for example, focusing on symptom remission, on quality of life, and on pharmacoeconomics) would also be useful for future GAD studies.

Dramatic advances in psychiatric methodologies should allow future developments in understanding the psychobiology of GAD. Molecular imaging, for example, is providing exciting opportunities for integrating neuroanatomical and neurochemical information about different psychiatric disorders. The completion of the human genome scan will provide many opportunities for understanding the neurogenetics of anxiety and other conditions. Second and third messenger systems are likely to provide important treatment targets in the future. Cognitive-affective neuroscience may ultimately allow an integration of biological findings with psychological research on worry processes and on underlying schemas.

One of the more immediately accessible issues in the drug treatment of GAD is how the antidepressants effective in GAD actually mediate their therapeutic benefit. It is well known that these medications take some time to work, and this delay has been attributed to the time needed to down-regulate presynaptic 5-HT autoreceptors. It is now possible to test this theory using imaging techniques with 5-HT_{1A} tracers such as 11C-WAY 100635. Additional questions concern whether down-regulation of presynaptic receptors results in increased synaptic 5-HT, or whether post-synaptic or downstream second messenger changes are more critical. Tryptophan depletion studies, for example, have been useful in suggesting that SSRI-induced increases in synaptic 5-HT are crucial in depression and panic, but perhaps less important in obsessive-compulsive disorder.[18,19] The application of such paradigms to GAD would seem timely.

In a similar context, recent work has shown that the antidepressant effects of noradrenergic antidepressants such as desipramine can be reversed by decreasing noradrenaline synthesis with α-methylparatyrozine.[20] In contrast, tryptophan depletion had no effect on the antidepressant action of such drugs. Venlafaxine is clearly effective in GAD and at doses over about 125mg a day is probably acting on the noradrenergic site as well as the serotonergic uptake one.[21] It would therefore be of some interest to see whether the therapeutic effect of GAD was sensitive both to tryptophan depletion and to noradrenaline depletion with α-methylparatyrozine.

Future work should address the question of how best to sequence and combine medications and psychotherapy in GAD. Direct head-to-head comparisons of newer agents are also needed. There is relatively little work on the effectiveness (as opposed to efficacy) of GAD treatment; showing that particular interventions are effective in patients with comorbid conditions and in everyday medical settings. There is also a relative dearth of studies on maintenance pharmacotherapy, on the treatment of refractory patients, and on the management of pediatric and geriatric GAD.

The question of whether early intervention for GAD will prevent psychiatric comorbidity (perhaps by affecting trait as well as state anxiety), reduce medical comorbidity, and improve long-term prognosis and disability is another exciting area for future investigation. Finally, the fact that placebo response in GAD is not only relatively high but also clinically significant deserves further study, both in order to help improve future interventions for GAD and to help reduce placebo response in future clinical trials.

Conclusion

The clinician can perhaps be forgiven for having been somewhat confused about GAD in the past. Diagnostic criteria for GAD have varied considerably from one edition to the next of the DSM, and differ between the DSM-IV and ICD-10. There has also been a lack of clarity about whether the disorder is a residual disorder (it is not), about whether it exists in a pure rather than comorbid form (it does), and about its defining characteristics (which may revolve more around psychic and somatic tension than worry). Additional confusing phenomena include the fact that prevalence is relatively low in comparision to the 10% figure for anxiety neurosis, that the psychobiology of GAD is not well understood, and that 'antidepressants' are effective for an anxiety condition.

Nevertheless, in recent years there has been growing clarity about GAD, with advances in understanding its phenomenology, pathogenesis, pharmacotherapy, and psychotherapy. We need to emphasize to our colleagues in primary care that GAD is independent, prevalent, persistent, and disabling. We need to emphasize that the more recently introduced antidepressants (SSRIs and SNRIs) as well as CBT are treatments of choice, and that these interventions are effective and well tolerated. We need to emphasize that while GAD patients can be demanding and frustrating, it is possible to build a supportive relationship that is rewarding for the clinician and helpful for the patient. Future refinements and advances in the field of GAD will further contribute to successful treatment of these patients.

References

1. Ormel J, Koeter MWJ, van den Brink W et al., Recognition, management, and course of anxiety and depression in general practice, *Arch Gen Psychiatry* (1991) 48:700–6

2. Stein DJ, Comorbidity in generalized anxiety disorder: Impact and implications, *J Clin Psychiatry* (2001) **62S**:29–36

3. Freud S, Collected papers, Vol I. (London: Hogarth Press, 1957) 76–106

4. Rickels K, Rynn MA, What is generalized anxiety disorder?, *J Clin Psychiatry* (2001) **62S11**:4–12

5. Carter RM, Wittchen H-U, Pfister H et al., One-year prevalence of subthreshold and threshold DSM-IV generalized anxiety disorder in a nationally representative sample, *Depress Anxiety* (2001) 3:78–88

6. Kessler RC, The epidemiology of pure and comorbid generalized anxiety disorder. A review and evaluation of recent research, *Acta Psychiatr Scand* (2001) 406 (Suppl):7–13

7. Kessler RC, Andrade L, Bijl RV et al., The effects of comorbidity on the onset and persistence of generalized anxiety disorder in the ICPE surveys 2001. (2002)

8. Maier W, Gansicke A, Freyberger HJ et al., Generalized anxiety disorder (ICD-10) in primary care from a cross-cultural perspective: a valid diagnostic entity?, *Acta Psychiatr Scand* (2000) 101: 29–36

9. Rickels K, Schweitzer E, Long-term treatment of anxiety disorders: maintenance treatment studies in anxiety disorders: some methodological notes, *Psychopharmacol Bull* (1995) 31:115–23

10. Wittchen H-U, Carter RM, Pfister H et al., Disabilities and quality of life in pure and comorbid generalized anxiety disorder and major depression in a national survey, *Int Clin Psychopharmacol* (2000) 15:319–28

11. Kirmayer LJ, Robbins JM, Dworkind M et al., Somatization and the recognition of depression and anxiety in primary care, *Am J Psychiatry* (1993) 150:734–41

12. Stein DJ, Hollander E, *Anxiety Disorders Comorbid with Depression: Social Anxiety Disorder, Post-traumatic Stress Disorder, Generalized Anxiety Disorder and Obsessive-Compulsive Disorder.* (London: Martin Dunitz, 2002)

13. Finlay-Jones R, Brown GW, Types of stressful life events and the onset of anxiety and depressive disorders, *Psychol Med* (1981) 11:803–15

14. Lin EH, Katon W, Von Korff M et al., Frustrating patients: physician and patient perspectives among distressed high users of medical services, *J Gen Intern Med* (1991) 6:241–6

15. Fawcett J, Stein DJ, Jobson KO, *Textbook of Treatment Algorithms in Psychopharmacology*, (Chichester: John Wiley & Sons, 1999)

16. Ballenger JC, Davidson JR, Lecrubier Y et al., Consensus statement on generalized anxiety disorder from the International Consensus Group on Depression and Anxiety, *J Clin Psychiatry* (2001) **62S11**:53–8

17. El-Khayat R, Baldwin DS, Antipsychotic drugs for non-psychotic patients: assessment of the benefit/risk ratio in generalized anxiety disorder, *J Psychopharmacol* (1998) 12:323–9

18. Bell C, Abrams J, Nutt DJ, Tryptophan depletion and its implications for psychiatry, *Br J Psychiatry* (2001) 178:399–405

19. Bell C, Forshall S, Adrover M, Nash J, Hood S, Argyropoulos S, Rich A, Nutt DJ, Does 5-HT restrain panic? A tryptophan depletion study in panic disorder patients recovered on paroxetine, *J Psychopharmacol* (2002) 16:5–14

20. Miller HL, Delgado PL, Salomon RM et al, Clinical and biochemical effects of catecholamines depletion on antidepressant-induced remission of depression, *Arch Gen Psychiatry* (1996) 53:117–28

21. Melichar JK, Haida A, Rhodes C, Reynolds AH et al., Venlafaxine occupation at the noradrenaline reuptake site: in vivo determination in healthy volunteers, *J Psychopharmacol* (2001) 15:9–12

Index

Note: Page numbers in **bold** refer to figures in the text; *italics* refer to tables or boxed material. (i) following a page reference indicates material in the footnotes.